Saving Amy

By

Janice Lawson

Published by
Creating-Design
P.O. Box 1785
Columbus, IN 47202

www.creating-design.com

"That I may publish with the voice of thanksgiving, and tell of all thy wondrous works." ~Psalms 26:7

Foreword

I first met the Lawson family when Amy was placed in my fifth grade class. Early in the school year, we had several conversations about special accommodations Amy needed due to some health problems. I don't think I fully grasped what they had been through due to the Lawsons as well as Amy being so determined to move forward.

It was when Michael contacted me to write a short article about his wife, Janice, and her care for Amy that I started realizing even more what they had experienced. Minnesota was their home for three years of their lives because Amy entered this world with a rare kidney disease and frequently required the services of University of Minnesota Hospital. During our conversation, I remembered thinking about how important it was for our two daughters to be healthy when born. They were with the exception of an eye problem that was corrected with one surgery!

Amy's problems were life threatening on more than one occasion. Janice, being her mom and a former nurse, found herself constantly doing every thing in her power to keep Amy alive. Doctors, other medical personnel, family members, friends, churches, and communities all gave tremendous efforts toward helping. While you are reading Janice's accounts of the journey to save Amy, you will get a real sense of the importance of her faith and the faith of Amy as well as others. Saving Amy is a book readers will want to finish once started, a book that will likely make most readers feel very fortunate, a book that will help some readers cope better with their own family health battles.

And, you will understand why when I asked fifth graders to do a plate for a Thanksgiving bulletin board that Amy did a plate with the following words, "I'm thankful for my life!"

David Webster

Contents

Chapter 1

The Birth

This is the story of my daughter, Amy, and her struggle for life. It is also the story of my struggle to find God in this battle.

Amy was born on April 13, 1983. The day started sunny and bright, but it was raining by the time Amy arrived at 6:16 p.m. As the nurse rubbed her with a towel, Amy peed. The nurse laughed and looked at her daddy saying, "At least we know her kidneys work."

Amy was finally placed in my arms. She looked at me as if knowing who I was, and I felt the first of a powerful rush of love for this tiny little creature. After what seemed a very short time, we were wheeled down the hall to my room. It wasn't long before Amy was taken from my arms. She immediately protested and cried out what sounded like "mama." The nurse smiled and said, "She's already calling for her mama."

The doctor pronounced her healthy. She was 6 pounds 15 ounces and 20 7/8 inches long. Her Apgar score was 8-10. The nurse explained this was good. It showed how well she was doing at birth. We had a beautiful and healthy little girl! Our only problem seemed to be in nursing, a latching problem. I was told not to worry, that first babies often have difficulty in the beginning. We stayed an extra day in the hospital to learn proper nursing techniques.

We took her home. She was three days old, and I was already feeling as if she had always existed. She was perfect! I never wanted to put her down. I enjoyed looking at those perfect little lips and nostrils that flared as she nursed and played with her perfect little fingers that wound around my finger and hung on tight. She had ten perfect little toes that curled while kissing them. I was in heaven, completely content for the first time in my life. I could do this forever, just holding this precious little girl and staring into her eyes. What was she thinking as she looked back?

While holding her, I thought about the dreams I had while pregnant. In the first dream, I am pregnant, but carrying the fetus around in a test tube. I hand the tube to Michael, but we somehow drop it. The tube hits the ground and shatters into many pieces. I frantically bend over the site to look, but all I see are particles scattered about that look like sugar crystals.

The second dream occurred about six months into the pregnancy. I am sitting on my living room sofa and have taken the baby out of my abdomen while letting the child move about the room still attached to what seems to be the umbilical cord.

Then, there was a third dream shortly before Amy was born. In that dream, the baby's bottom is on fire, and Michael is trying to put it out but can't. I suddenly grab the child, run to the bathroom and place her (or him) into the sink which is filled with water extinguishing the fire.

The dreams were quite bothersome. What if they were a premonition of something being wrong with the baby? I told my friend, Katie, about the dreams. She laughed and assured me that every pregnant mother has strange silly dreams about her baby.

As I held Amy in my arms, I knew the dreams were definitely just that-strange silly dreams. She was perfect, not a single thing wrong.

Then, the crying started. She was two or three weeks old and seemed to cry 24 hours a day. When Michael came home from work, I would hand her to him the moment he walked in the door. She would be screaming; I would be crying.

"Do something!" I would beg him. "She won't stop crying." He would put her high on his shoulder and waltz around the living room. She would quiet down for a while, and then he would bring her to me.

"She's hungry," he would tell me as he placed her beside me. I would offer my breast, and she would attach hungrily and nurse. Before long, she would abruptly stop and begin to cry as her little feet would attempt to climb up me. I would pull her back down and help her reattach. We would repeat the cycle over and over until it seemed she was full. She was getting plenty of milk; so, what was wrong? Why did she act in this bizarre way?

When she was four weeks old, I went to my family doctor for my postpartum checkup. He delivered her and would continue caring for her. I told him our baby cried almost all the time. He suggested, with a smile on his face, that's what babies do! No, I stressed it was excessive and wondered if it could be colic. He seemed to dismiss my concerns and would see her in a couple of weeks for the six-week exam.

I left the office depressed and on the verge of tears. I felt so inadequate! Being a nurse, we listened to the doctor. I would just deal with it. It must be colic. She seemed okay when not screaming and trying to climb while nursing. Her smile melted us! She knew my arms. Even if I gave her to someone else when asleep, she would awaken and cry until I took her back.

Despite all the fussing and crying, I was falling deeper and deeper in love with her. I had heard of people shaking or throwing their babies when they couldn't get the crying to stop. How could that happen? I just held her closer and cried right along with her!

During the week that Amy was to see the doctor for her six-week checkup, she began to vomit. Feeding had become a nightmare! The regular problems with eating, crying, screaming and kicking her feet were now joined with vomiting. I was getting worried. Her little face had broken out in a red and slightly raised rash. I was anxious for the doctor to see her.

The day of the appointment, Michael had to work. We were down to one car. Amy and I had to take the city bus. I worried about her vomiting on the bus. The appointment was at the time she normally napped which meant I would not get my resting period. I was quite exhausted!

She slept through the appointment. At six weeks of age, she only weighed 7 pounds 3 ounces, a gain of less than four ounces since birth. The doctor was concerned about her weight. He believed my breast milk wasn't nutritious enough. I was to stop nursing and to try cans of a formula.

He examined her face and gave me a prescription for an ointment. She might have colic, and he gave me another prescription. While examining her, he asked if she always slept so soundly. I stressed it was not typical at all even though it

4

was her naptime. He didn't seem concerned and gave me the name of another formula if she continued to vomit. Then, he was gone! The nurse ushered us out of the exam room.

I left the building and trudged across the street holding Amy close and wondering how I would manage on the bus with her, a diaper bag, my purse and now cans of formula. I felt confused; the doctor hadn't seemed to address the exact problem. What the problem was, I did not know. I did know something was not right with my baby!

Michael decided a vacation might be helpful. He would take me, Amy and my 15 year old sister, Lorena, who lived with us to Tulsa, Oklahoma to visit my oldest brother, Elton. The trip there was uneventful. We stopped several times during the drive to see different sights. Amy slept much of the trip. The vomiting was somewhat better. Perhaps, the formula was the answer. I felt miserable; I couldn't even nurse my baby; my milk wasn't good enough!

In Tulsa, we stayed with my brother, his wife and their 18 month old son. Lita was pregnant with their second son. I was happy to show off my daughter but wished she looked healthier. I don't remember much about the trip; Amy was constantly on my mind. Something still didn't seem right. I could remember visiting Oral Roberts University, but I couldn't remember anything about it shortly afterwards.

On the second night there, I was in bed with Amy attempting to get her to eat. She just cried and cried. My brother came into the room wondering what was wrong. He commented that she cried an awful lot compared to his son and left the room. Suddenly, Amy started choking. She stopped crying, and her color became dark. I raised her up, and she made a strange noise. The most horrible feeling overwhelmed me. I didn't know what was happening; something terrible was wrong with my baby! I slept that night with her cradled in my arms.

The next day, I told Michael we should go home because Amy needed to see the doctors. Once home, I called the doctor to report Amy was not keeping either formula down. I was to switch her to a soybean formula and to start her on baby food. It was my opinion that it was too soon for baby food, but I followed the doctor's orders. She did not keep the soy formula down any better. The baby food also came back up. It was supposed to stay down since it was thicker than formula. It not only didn't stay down, the thickness caused her to become choked every time she vomited. I was scared!

Chapter 2

Admission to Hospital

On Saturday, July 9, I looked at my baby and saw death. Her eyes no longer sparkled; they looked clouded over; her cry was weak. She saw a different doctor earlier in the week. He picked up on nothing and sent us home with just another change in formula. We felt she was getting worse and took her to the emergency room.

The doctor examined her. She had lost three ounces in the last two days, but he didn't seem too concerned. I asked if he didn't think that was too much for a little infant to lose. He looked straight at me and said, "Well, yes, but she isn't going to die from it. Take her to her doctor on Monday."

He discharged her from ER without doing anything when I thought it was time to keep her for more tests. She was so sick that she could barely cry. I was up all Saturday night with her. At 5:00 Sunday morning, I told Michael we had to take her back to the emergency room.

Upon arriving, we discovered the same doctor was still on duty. I turned to Michael and stressed we needed our own doctor. When the other one entered the exam room, Michael requested our family doctor. When Amy's doctor arrived, he took one look at her and called in a pediatrician and admitted her to the hospital.

I felt a little hope rise up and could relax a little. Somebody else was taking over. They would find out what was making my baby ill and fix her. She would be fine.

Amy was admitted to the Pediatric Unit with the diagnosis of "failure to thrive." I was crushed. I had worked the Pediatric Unit and knew what was being whispered quietly among the nurses. A failure to thrive diagnosis usually meant failure of the parents. Here I was, a nurse, and could not even get my own baby to thrive.

Shortly after arriving in Amy's room, a nurse came in with a bottle of formula. I reached for it, but the nurse pulled it away. Taking Amy from my arms, she was going to feed my baby. She sat down holding Amy in a semi-upright position and offered her the nipple. Amy's little lips closed down around the nipple and began to drink. I told the nurse Amy would vomit. The nurse explained how a baby had to have her head raised and be fed slowly.

Michael and I just looked at each other. Did she think we were idiots? She believed Amy had problems because we didn't know how to feed her. She fed Amy about an ounce, and she didn't vomit. The nurse stood up, handed my baby back and instructed me not to feed her at all. She would be back in a while to give her more. Michael and I didn't know what to say to each other.

The pediatrician arrived and didn't even touch Amy. He looked at her and then said something that really scared me, "That is a very sick little baby." He left the room after telling us he was ordering some tests.

Later, a lab technician came in and performed a test for cystic fibrosis. I watched as she placed a small cup over the skin on Amy's lower arm and waited for her to sweat under it. Then, she swabbed the area. It would take several days to get the results. I knew something was wrong with my baby, but I didn't think she had cystic fibrosis.

Another technician arrived to draw blood from Amy. The technician had to stick Amy's little heels many times to get enough blood. She cried the entire time as the woman stuck and squeezed and squeezed more. Her cry was so weak. I felt so helpless! I couldn't tell the woman to stop; we had to know what was wrong. One thing was for certain, Amy was not thriving because of our lack of parenting skills! Something terrible was wrong, and we had to know what was attacking her little body.

While waiting for the results, Michael decided we both needed to eat. I couldn't remember when I actually had eaten. He left the hospital and returned with a hamburger for each of us. I ate the sandwich as I watched Amy sleep. She looked so pale. Her face was still broken out in that strange rash, and her breathing didn't seem right. Amy did not look like the baby I had given birth to just eleven weeks earlier. It had been a long, difficult eight weeks between the worsening of the vomiting, the lack of weight gain and all the trips to the doctor. I was exhausted and probably suffering from postpartum depression along with the stress of the entire situation.

A couple of hours after the blood draws, the nurse returned to the room. I needed to come to the nurses' station because the pediatrician was on the phone. Once there, the doctor explained that the test results were back, and they showed Amy was in complete kidney failure. I went into shock.

"Both kidneys?" I asked. The answer was yes. Her creatinine was 8.5, normal results were about 0.5; her BUN was 222, normal was under 20. These were two of the tests that showed kidney failure.

He continued to talk, but I was missing most of what he was saying. How could this be happening? My mother, grandmother and great-grandmother had all died of kidney problems. How could this have skipped me and attacked my baby? I felt dizzy, nauseated and unable to breathe. But, I had to listen; my baby's life depended on it! I heard him speak horrible words-kidney failure, death, nothing could be done. She was being transferred to the children's hospital in Indianapolis.

The doctor asked if Michael and I could take her there immediately. They could send her by ambulance; however, there wasn't anything paramedics could do, and the ambulance was needed at the hospital. He stressed again the importance of taking her immediately. Her potassium level was at 2.5. If it dropped to 2.4, she would go into cardiac arrest. He estimated she had six hours to live.

I handed the phone back to the nurse to get the order for transfer. I stumbled back to the room, tears streaming down my face. Michael met me at the door. He wanted to know what the doctor had said. All I could manage to say was "kidney failure."

I gathered my sweet little baby up in my arms. This can't be happening. My brother and sister have healthy children. Why isn't my baby healthy? What horrible thing have I done that my baby deserves this? Questions such as these ran over and over through my mind as the nurse made arrangements.

Michael gathered up our things. It seemed all of a sudden that the nurse, Amy and I were at the exit door waiting for Michael to bring the car. Standing there, I asked the nurse how much of a chance she felt Amy had of living.

She answered, "I don't know, but if anything can be done, it will be done there." She was referring to Riley Children's Hospital. The sickest children from all over the state were at this hospital, even children from other states.

In 1983, Riley Hospital was a very old building located in a very shabby part of Indianapolis. The neighborhood, at that time, consisted of many abandoned dilapidated buildings. Winos and other homeless men were sleeping in the doorways and openly on the sidewalks. Women, apparently prostitutes, were standing on the street corners. Groups of scary looking young men were huddled together. I stared out the window wondering what kind of place we were bringing our child for help.

Amy vomited several times during the trip, thanks to the feeding the nurse had forced earlier I thought. I cleaned her as well as possible and prayed the entire trip. I felt as if I were in a nightmare and couldn't wake up, but I was fortunate that I could not foresee the rest of the nightmare and the torture my baby would have to endure.

Sitting in the vehicle beside my ill baby, I wondered if God was punishing me for ignoring Him and not attending church ever since my parents stopped taking me.

Chapter 3

Finding a Diagnosis

I was raised in a very strict church. It was a frightening experience, especially for a shy, little girl. The minister would jump up and down, scream and point his finger at someone and tell them they were a sinner and God was going to strike them down. I would crouch down in the pew and hope I wasn't the one about to get struck down. People would dance around the pews, yelling and speaking strange words that I didn't understand.

We were not allowed to listen to secular music, watch TV, wear shorts, cut our hair, wear make-up, dance, etc. It seemed to me we pretty much couldn't do anything.

I remember being about four years old and having one of my many ear infections. I had fallen asleep on one of the pews. My mother must have asked the minister to pray for me because I awoke to find several people standing over me, their hands on me. They were talking in very loud voices. I squeezed my eyes shut and hoped God was not about to strike me down.

My parents quit taking us there; I can't remember why. We would occasionally go somewhere else but were never actual members of any church. Due to the things I had experienced, I thought God was out to get us. My mother, though, was a true believer in God and was able to teach me that God would take care of us.

When I was 17, my boyfriend took me to his church. This Christian church was huge and quite different from that little church of my early childhood. In June of 1974 at the age of 18, I was baptized in that church in front of at least 300 people. I accepted Jesus Christ as my Savior but seldom attended church over the next nine years.

Before Amy was born, Michael and I started attending Garden City Church of Christ even though it was hit and miss, mainly miss for me due to working the night shift. When I got off work at 7 a.m., bed sounded better than a church pew.

The thought that God was punishing me kept running through my head, but deep inside, even with my lack of Bible knowledge, I knew God would not do that to me. God was a good God. My mother had taught me about His goodness. He loved my baby, probably even more than I did.

When we arrived at the hospital ER, we were rushed in. Papers had to be filled out and signed. We were told the nephrologists had been called and would arrive soon. Indeed, they arrived quickly. Dr. Bergstein was a very tall, older gentleman. His partner, Dr. Sharon Andreoli, was a younger female doctor.

They stated it was rare for an infant to go into kidney failure after birth. Amy was very ill, very near death. Her potassium blood level that morning in the Columbus hospital was so low that she needed to be on IV potassium without delay. It was critical to find out what had caused her kidney to fail to determine if the failure could be reversed.

The doctors asked questions about Amy's birth, how she had been those first two weeks after her birth and how her condition had deteriorated over the next nine weeks. We were questioned about other family members. I shared that my mother died at the age of 49 after surgery for a probable malignant kidney. My grandmother and great-grandmother also died of some type of kidney disease in their 60's, but I did not know any details.

Amy was taken for an x-ray of her kidneys before being admitted to intensive care. Afterward, Dr. Andreoli explained that Amy's kidneys could be seen on the x-ray. This was not supposed to happen. She only knew of one disease that make them visible. It was Hyperoxaluria, a very rare genetic disease, one that caused oxalate crystals to accumulate in the body causing first kidney failure and then other problems. It also just happened that Dr. Andreoli had joined Riley recently. She had been at the University of Minnesota training under a doctor researching this disease. It was the only hospital offering help and kidney transplants for patients with this rare disease.

She suspected Amy had oxalosis, as this disease was also called, but she would have to perform a biopsy to know for sure. Later, Michael and I would marvel at God's plans that placed this doctor right where we needed her when we needed her.

Amy was admitted to the Intensive Care Unit, and we were left in the waiting room while the doctor worked to save her life. Michael paced the floor, and I collapsed in a chair to cry and attempt to understand why this was happening. But, there was not any understanding! I wanted to scream at God for allowing this horrible disease but was too frightened. If I did, would He go ahead and take my child as my punishment?

"Lord, why did you give me this wonderful baby and fill my heart and soul with so much love for her if you are going to take her?" I asked. There was no answer, only silence.

Someone came to get us. They explained Amy was now on peritoneal dialysis. She was attached to all kinds of tubes and equipment. Walking into the small room, I almost collapsed. As a nurse, I had witnessed patients in all kinds of conditions, but nothing compared to what I saw then. Amy was strapped down in a crib. She could not move anything but her head. This was necessary, the doctor explained, because she could not disrupt the catheter that entered through an incision in her tiny abdomen. The catheter was positioned between the walls of the abdomen in an area called the peritoneal cavity. A special solution would be inserted and left creating a space. It would be left there for a certain amount of time to absorb waste products and fluid that her kidneys were no longer removing. Then, the solution would be removed, discarded and replaced. This would be repeated over and over until her blood levels were as close to normal as possible. The catheter had been sutured to her skin and extended through the bottom of an upside down foam cup which was taped to her abdomen to help prevent disruption of the catheter.

Another catheter went into her bladder to drain urine, but there wasn't any urine. An IV line had been placed in a vein in her head; the hair had been shaved around the area. Potassium was being dripped in to raise her potassium level out of the danger level. Heart monitors had been attached to her tiny chest, and an oximeter had been clipped and taped to a tiny finger to monitor oxygen levels. It was difficult to see among all the machines and tubes that there was a tiny little baby in that crib, my baby!

Throughout the next 48 hours, we were allowed ten minute visits every hour. For the remaining 50 minutes, we did not know what was happening with our baby. Was she still alive? Was she tolerating the procedures? Were all the treatments doing what the doctors hoped they would? So, every hour we struggled down a long hall, turned a corner and would enter the Intensive Care Unit. We would go into the room and pray that Amy was doing well. Her personal nurse, sitting at her bedside, would give us the past hour report-how things were going, how Amy was tolerating everything and what was expected in the next hour.

Amy slept, moaned and cried. She would not open her eyes. I touched and kissed the only available spot on her tiny little forehead. Michael would take his turn. Afterward, we would walk back down the hall together to wait for the next visit. This went on all night. By morning, I could barely walk but kept going. It was the only way I could see that my baby was still alive.

Once Amy's kidney waste levels were lowered enough, the dialysis would be stopped. She would be observed in hopes her kidneys might start functioning again. Sometimes it happened. However, if Amy did have oxalosis, function would never return, and she would need a kidney transplant. Amy would need to weigh 20 pounds to receive a kidney transplant. It might take two years for her to gain enough weight since children in kidney failure gained weight very slowly. Dr. Andreoli stressed that time for these children was extremely critical.

Oxalosis is a condition in which the liver is missing an enzyme needed to break down oxalate in the human body. Without the enzyme, oxalate crystals accumulate in the body, not only destroying the kidneys but also building up in other body organs and the retina of the eyes causing blindness. I asked about damage to the other organs such as the heart and liver when this occurred. This was unknown because no one had lived long enough for this to be determined.

The words cut through me sharper than a knife. My God, how could this be happening? This diagnosis seemed to be a definite death sentence! There was no way even to know until Amy had stabilized enough to have surgery to obtain the kidney tissue for biopsy.

I had not been in church enough or read the Bible to have much knowledge of what God could do, but I did know He could heal. I began to pray for a miraculous healing for my little baby. Amy had suffered enough already. In the past two days, she had endured more torture than most people in their lifetime. It was now clearer how much Amy had suffered the last two months. We had assumed she had colic as the doctor suggested. She had continued to have wet diapers right up until her hospital admission. This was possible, stated Dr. Andreoli, due to a condition called high urine output kidney failure.

I could hardly bear all the thoughts! No wonder she always cried and spent most of her time kicking her legs. Perhaps, as in my dream, she felt she was on fire. I would have gladly taken all her suffering upon myself if it had just been possible. I wanted my baby well! Where are you, God? I demanded to know! Please, heal my baby. How blessed we are that we cannot sell our soul to satan because that's what I would have done at that time to see my baby well.

Over the first 48 hours of dialysis, Amy's little body started absorbing the fluid. Her body became bloated as she gained several pounds. She looked horrible. Her skin was stretched with an appearance that made everyone cringe. The doctors didn't have any answers as to why. Dr. Andreoli called the University of Minnesota Hospital hoping to find an answer. There was none. Our worry went from cardiac failure due to low potassium to cardiac failure due to fluid overload.

On Tuesday, Michael insisted I go home and rest. He would call if anything changed and would continue to visit her every hour. I couldn't possibly rest and didn't want to be over an hour away, but he kept insisting. I decided to go home, take a shower, change clothing and check on things.

I cried the whole drive home. When I arrived home, my sister Shirley was there. She had come to stay with our younger sister, Lorena, while I was at the hospital. Shirley had her own 18-month-old baby, Lauren, and a friend's baby with her.

I must have looked pretty bad from the expression on Shirley's face. Wherever I looked in the apartment, I saw evidence of Amy-the bassinet, the box of diapers beside it and her toys still scattered about. How I longed for her to be back home, but I knew it wouldn't be any time soon. I started toward the bedroom. My sister followed.

"Do you want me to take the babies somewhere else?" she asked. I knew she realized that their presence might make me even sadder.

"No," I told her; "I won't be here long."

I closed the door, turned on the shower and began removing my clothing. As I removed my shirt, I noticed my bra was becoming wet. This would develop when nursing Amy if I was a little late, but I hadn't nursed her for weeks. My milk had dried up. Removing my bra, I saw clear liquid running from my breasts. They looked like tear drops. It was as if my body was crying for my baby left behind at the hospital.

Chapter 4

Our Lives Completely Change

Thursday seemed no better than Sunday when we brought Amy to Riley Hospital. We were exhausted, hardly getting any sleep while staying in the waiting room keeping our hourly ten-minute vigil. It was the only way we knew what was developing from hour to hour with our precious baby.

I roamed the halls of the old hospital between visits. It was my first time for being in a children's hospital; my nurses training hadn't included that experience. I was heartbroken at the sights. Sick children were everywhere, many on the verge of death. The ill children I had been exposed to were in the hospital for pneumonia, tonsillectomies, ear tubes or other minor procedures. Now, I was seeing children with deformed limbs and signs of cancer such as bald heads, sunken eyes and toting IV poles.

I saw a nurse pushing a child in a wheelchair. The body looked like a very scrawny two-year-old child, but the head was three times the size of my own. Little eyes peered out from the massive face. A restraint was around the child's forehead tying the head in place. If released, the large head would topple over and cause the child's neck to break.

My God, my mind screamed, why is there such a need for a place like this? Why don't you heal these pitiful little children I cried while working my way through the halls back to my own little one?

"God, please let Amy live. Show me a sign so I'll have hope and know You are listening and know You are with her."

On schedule, Michael and I went to visit Amy. She looked the same-bloated, strapped down, whimpering at times and surrounded by tubing attached to her everywhere. Even with all of Amy's crying since birth, I had seen a happy child. Amy started smiling during her first month of life. She would stare into my eyes as I talked and actually smile! I wanted so much to see that smile again. For days now, I had not seen anything of her personality. She had been and still was so close to death. Were we going to lose her after falling so deeply in love?

I bent over her, and she turned her head toward me. I kissed her forehead and repeatedly expressed how much I loved her and how much I wanted to hold her. Suddenly, she opened her eyes briefly and smiled. My heart leaped. Amy would leave this little room alive! I felt God in that room for the first time; I had my sign from Him!

Two days later, the doctors removed the dialysis tube and transferred her to the Infant Care Unit. I could hold her again, love on her, kiss her and watch her expressions as I talked.

Amy's kidneys would be carefully watched. If function didn't return, a permanent peritoneal dialysis catheter would be inserted and dialysis would resume. They could wait about a week to perform the procedure if her condition remained stable.

The infant unit was a very large open room. The nurses' station was at the front of the room with crib upon crib lined in rows across the room. At each crib, there was a recliner where a parent could sit and sleep, if possible, in the noisy active room. Nurses reported to each other and the doctors, babies cried, machines beeped and a host of other noises were constant. At least, I could sit in the recliner and hold my precious baby encouraging her to get better.

Since the room was open, any contagious infection in one baby soon spread to another. Upon Amy's arrival in the unit, a severe intestinal bacterium, C-Diff, was on the rampage. It moved from baby to baby, causing severe diarrhea resulting in dehydration and other problems. Small babies could die quickly from this disease. Michael and I were worried. We inquired about a private room, but they didn't exist. We felt Amy's weak body could not fight off this infection if she were to catch it. How could we protect her? We couldn't!

Along with this worry, we were informed Amy had been exposed to chicken pox by a medical student. The medical staff was in an uproar. Should Amy break out in chicken pox, which could happen soon, it would spread throughout the unit. What more could happen, we wondered? Amy wouldn't survive either illness!

The staff met and informed us, due to the circumstances, Amy would be moved into the isolation room. It was the only private room, which earlier hadn't existed on the unit. The other babies would be protected from chicken pox, problem solved. What the staff didn't realize was that God was protecting Amy!

We were seeing the beginning of many miracles throughout Amy's struggle for good health. In the tiny little private room, I was able to sleep when she did. Michael and I stayed close by 24/7. He slept in a waiting room, and I slept on a cot beside Amy's crib. She did not develop C-Diff, chicken pox or any other lurking infections.

Over the next week, we prayed for a miracle. We needed Amy's kidney function to return. God was there. We knew her kidneys would resume the job they had been designed to do. However, day after day, the laboratory reports proved that was not the case. She was still in kidney failure.

The doctors took her to surgery. A peritoneal dialysis catheter was placed back in her abdomen, and a tiny slice of her kidney was removed for biopsy. The results would be available a few days later. I was devastated! My baby was attached to a catheter tubing approximately five feet long which was connected to a bag of solution that would keep her alive. Michael and I would be trained how to administer the dialysis, and we would take Amy home to await a kidney transplant.

My friend, Katie, came to visit. We were sitting in Amy's room chatting when suddenly she said, "Janice, look at my arm." Katie had goose bumps all over her arm while picking up Amy's dialysis tubing and holding it up.

"This is your cord from your second dream." I looked at the tube and had a sudden feeling of déjà vu. Could this have been the meaning of my dream?

When the biopsy results returned, Amy was officially diagnosed as having hyperoxaluria. Dr. Andreoli discussed how it was a rare genetic disease. Amy had received a defective gene from both of us.

I could not understand how this had happened. If this was such a rare gene, then what were the chances of Michael and I both having it? Even then, Amy had only a 25% chance of having the disease. I had never heard of this disease. My brother and sister each had a child, and their children were healthy. Why did this happen to us, to Amy? I wanted to be angry, but who could I be angry with, perhaps God? He had allowed it, didn't he? Yet, I was too frightened to be angry with God. I didn't know Him well enough to know how He would handle it. Maybe He would take Amy from me. This I knew was something I could not bear.

Getting from the start of dialysis to receiving a kidney transplant was going to be a long and difficult journey. She barely weighed seven pounds. Indiana University Medical Center was performing kidney transplants on children in 1983. However, they had to weigh 20 pounds, and the center had never successfully performed a kidney transplant on a child with oxalosis.

As long as Amy was in kidney failure, the oxalate crystals would continue to accumulate in her body causing more damage, such as blindness. She needed a functioning kidney immediately, but we were a long way from the 20 pound requirement. We were in a deep, dark hole. How were we to help Amy?

We took our baby home along with her five-foot-long tubing that would help us keep her alive for another day. That was how we lived, do what we had to for each day to keep Amy alive and healthy for another day. Our hope was at that 20 pound mark!

Michael returned to work. He had to keep money coming in and the insurance so Amy could receive what she needed medically. Each morning when Amy and I got up, I would drain the fluid from her abdomen into the bag attached to the tubing. While the fluid drained, I fed her a special high calorie formula which was to help with weight gain. To this formula, I added various medicines. She was unable to eat while the dialysis fluid remained between the abdominal walls. I would leave the fluid out for an hour while she ate and digested the formula and then change the bag and run new fluid back in.

Changing the bag was a major process all on its own. I would place Amy on the bed. The bag with its fluid and waste products that had been drawn off her tiny body would be on the dresser. I would have to turn off the furnace. If the furnace came on while I was changing the bag, the fan might cause air particles to enter the new bag and cause peritonitis.

Peritonitis was an infection that could occur in the walls of the abdomen. This infection would cause almost immediate illness and death if not promptly treated. In order to prevent this from occurring, many other precautions had to be in place. I had to wear a mask, and Amy's head had to be covered with a receiving blanket. She was too young for a mask; so, the blanket was to keep her from breathing, sneezing or coughing on the sterile part of the tubing as I changed it. I then had to scrub my hands with a special soap for three minutes. Afterwards, I would scrub the opening port of the old bag with an antibacterial solution, remove the protective covering from the new bag, take the catheter from the old bag and attach it to the new one. Then, a new sterile cap would be placed over the catheter where it attached to the bag. Once this was accomplished, I could remove my mask and Amy's blanket from her head. Amy was such a good baby. She seemed to understand her face needed to be covered and would not cry through the procedure, patiently waiting for it to end.

Once that was done, I would pick her and the bag up and move to the sofa. There, I would slowly run the fluid back into her abdomen. If we were both careful and lucky, Amy would not vomit her meal up as the fluid expanded her abdomen. This procedure was done four to five times a day from 7 a.m. until 9 p.m. The entire procedure took two to two and a half hours, a total of up to 12-13 hours a day, every day. The skin, where the catheter entered her abdomen, had to be cleansed. An antibiotic ointment was then applied followed by a new bandage. Most of the day was spent completing medical procedures.

Even with all the careful and slow movements, Amy would vomit three to six times a day. She and I lived in sweat pants and shirts. They were easy to peel off and throw in the washer. She always managed to vomit all over both of us every time!

Once a week, we would spend a day traveling to the Riley Hospital Clinic. The doctors would examine Amy, weigh her, draw her blood, change her medicine orders, her formula and adjust her dialysis solution. I would report to them how she was doing, how her feedings and dialysis procedures were going. They would in turn let me know what I needed to do next. The doctors were wonderful! Amy was doing great, and she was their pet project. They didn't know what we were doing right, but instructed us to keep it up because she was doing better than expected. We were praying. That's what we were doing!

Hardly a minute went by that I wasn't praying for Amy. Unfortunately, I forgot to pray for myself. I was a mess; I was exhausted! Amy was my 24-hour patient. I didn't do anything but care for my special little angel. I wouldn't have it any other way. Amy was mine; God had given her to me; I would care for her every minute of every day. This determination sent my 10-year struggle with depression into a downward spiral for the next 25 years.

Chapter 5

The Daily Struggle

The struggle for Amy to gain weight was endless. She needed a perfectly functioning kidney to protect her little body from the disease. Since she was in kidney failure, the oxalosis was still attacking her organs, her bones, her eyes, everything. The longer she was in kidney failure, the more damage was being done to her body. At the same time, she couldn't have a transplant until she weighed 20 pounds. It seemed to be a hopeless, endless cycle. She couldn't eat much; therefore, she couldn't gain a lot of weight. Without the weight, there could not be a transplant.

We lived on prayer! Somewhere I had heard the scripture that said, "Where two or more gather in my name, I will answer their prayer."

These were the words of Jesus; it must be true. Well, I reasoned, Amy and I were two. I would hold her close and tell her to believe with me for her healing. She would smile, reach up and pat my face.

Amy's first year of life revolved around her medical care. The doctor had warned us that Amy would develop peritonitis at some point. It was unavoidable! We knew exactly what to watch for and what to do when it happened. At the first symptom, we were to call the doctor and head to the hospital emergency room without any delay.

I was caring for Amy one day when realizing something just wasn't right; I knew Amy as well as I knew myself. When raising her shirt and feeling her little belly, it felt warm, kind of feverish. Then, I grabbed the clamp that kept the dialysis fluid in Amy's belly and pushed it open so the fluid could drain out. Panic struck! I hadn't seen it yet, but there it was now-a cloudy fluid, the horrible sign of peritonitis. I called the doctor, and she told me to bring her to the hospital-NOW! The hospital was an hour away, and Michael was at work with our only car, also an hour away. We couldn't delay two hours. I silently cursed myself for not having a plan for this situation, but I had hoped we would never see this day. Suddenly, for some unexplainable reason, I remembered a friend, another nurse, who lived in the same apartment complex. I called her about our predicament. She dropped everything, grabbed her kids, picked Amy and me up and took us to the hospital where Michael met us.

Amy was admitted and started on antibiotics. The hospital stay was rough. Amy was very ill the first 24 hours; she couldn't eat and hurt really bad. The only way she was comfortable was for me to sit very still and hold her with her belly against mine. While sitting in the chair, I could not move without causing her more pain. So, movement was impossible for me. I leaned my head back against the chair and closed my eyes. I would do anything for this little baby, but why God, why did she have to suffer? Opening my eyes, I was looking at a spot just above the doorway of the room. A banner was hanging there that read, "Trust the Lord with all your heart, and do not rely on your own understanding." (Proverbs 3:5)

My understanding of this entire situation with Amy was knowing we were helpless. I had never felt so sad, so alone. Where was God? Without a transplant quickly, we were losing the battle against the disease. I did the only thing I could do by placing all my trust in the hands of Jesus. Why do we need to reach that point before we turn to Him?

Over the next week, Amy regained her strength. The antibiotics seemed to be helping. But, as the doctors tested her dialysis fluid waste, the bacteria that caused the peritonitis continued to grow out in the cultures. She could not go home until the cultures were clear. The nurses watched our technique for changing the bags. A reason for the bacteria growth could not be determined; we were not accidentally contaminating the specimen! Finally, the doctor decided to send Amy to surgery to replace the catheter entering her body. Perhaps, that's where the contamination was coming from.

Once the catheter was replaced, the cultures returned negative. Amy was free of the bacteria! However, the entire stay had taken its toll on her. She had stopped eating and had lost weight. We were further behind schedule than ever! Before long, she resumed eating, eating and vomiting I should say.

Until this time, I had handled the feeding and vomiting problems. Amy had been gaining weight, just slowly. The doctors had been pleased. Even though her weight gain was slow, it was wonderful for a child in kidney failure.

Because of all the setbacks, the doctors considered a surgery that Michael and I did not want her to undergo, Nissan fundoplication. This surgery would tighten the sphincter between Amy's esophagus and stomach. The vomiting would be stopped, but then Amy would never be able to vomit again. What if her stomach hurt; what if in the future she swallowed something and needed to vomit? I didn't want her to have the surgery. We had been fighting against it since the beginning of her illness. Now, the doctors were telling us they felt it was medically necessary, perhaps even to save her life. They gave us until morning to give an answer.

Michael and I discussed it. We didn't know what to do. Michael finally left the decision to me. He felt I understood the procedure better, and I was the one who had to deal with her medical conditions the most. He kissed us good night and went home; I was sure to worry about it all night.

I gathered Amy into my arms, stared into those little brown eyes and asked what she thought. For six months, we had been struggling to keep her alive and to the point where she could have the kidney transplant enabling both of us to really live. I was exhausted, physically and emotionally. It was so unbearable at times, the struggle to get Amy to eat, only to have her vomit the entire meal. The physical trauma of vomiting that she endured was more than I could emotionally endure. The only thing that kept me going was knowing Amy needed me. If she wasn't going to give up, then I certainly could not either.

As I sat there in the chair holding her, crying and begging God to tell me what to do, Amy reached her little hand up and gently rubbed it against my cheek. She seemed to say, "It's okay mama. Whatever you decide, I will be fine."

I grabbed her little hand and brought it to my lips as tears spilled down and covered it. I kissed the hand and pulled her closer and began to sing *"Jesus Loves Me."* She looked at me and smiled that precious smile seemingly reserved for me and her daddy.

"Okay God, I guess I'm on my own on this decision."

Oh, how wrong our thoughts can be! I would learn that God was with us at that moment and continued to be every step of our journey.

As the doctors made their rounds the following morning, they again questioned me about the surgery. I agreed to it, and plans were started with the surgery scheduled for later in the week.

Since this was an abdominal surgery, Amy's peritoneal dialysis would have to be stopped. She would remain off dialysis until the surgery site healed. But, how was she to stay alive without dialysis? What if the healing took longer than expected? Children in kidney failure didn't heal well. What had I agreed to?

Amy only weighed about 9 pounds 8 ounces, and Riley Hospital did not have a lot of experience in hemodialysis of a small infant at that time. Hemodialysis is the machine that takes blood out of a patient's body, cleanses it and returns it to the patient. Just getting enough blood out of an infant's body to start the process was more blood than probably in their entire body.

I wasn't the only one worried. The doctors and nurses had to come up with a plan to make this work. If the plan failed, it would mean Amy's death. With all these plans going on around her, Amy wasn't worried! She was out of pain, no fevers, no traumatic events seem to be occurring. She appeared happy and enjoyed riding in the wagon as I pulled her about the hospital.

The night before the surgery, the surgeon visited. She was the same surgeon that had replaced the dialysis catheter the previous week. Now, she would be taking Amy to surgery again. As she examined Amy and chit-chatted about the surgery, she commented on how really good Amy looked as well as the skin around the new dialysis catheter. When removing the dressing from the old surgery site, her expression quickly changed. She asked how long the site had looked like this. Puzzled, I moved closer to the crib. The surgery site was red with drainage dripping from the incision. The surgeon pulled on a pair of gloves and pulled the incision apart. I thought I might faint. Nasty, thick drainage poured out. It had not looked like that the day before. Ripping off the gloves, she threw them in the trash along with the dressing.

"I cannot take that child to surgery in the morning; I'll have the nurse redress it."

I stared down at the incision. How did it get that bad so quickly? Throughout the next hour, people kept coming in to check Amy's incision. Nurses, her doctor and an infectious disease doctor all examined it. An antibiotic was ordered and quickly started. I called Michael and let him know the surgery had been canceled.

Over the next few days, Amy did well. No fevers from the infection and no other new problems were discovered. Since surgery was not an option any longer due to the infection, I begged the doctor to let me take her home. I could do the dialysis, antibiotics and dressing changes there. We could also work on the feeding problems at home just as well as in the hospital. The doctor agreed, but I had to bring her back to the clinic in a few days.

Amy began to eat better at home and started gaining weight. The incision healed up and became her best looking tummy scar. On one of her clinic visits, the doctor handed her back and once more told me to continue what we were doing because Amy looked wonderful and was doing great. I didn't tell her, but it wasn't us. Our church and most of the town of Columbus was praying!

While I was dealing with the daily rituals of keeping Amy alive and healthy, Michael began to speak with different people concerning Amy and the financial obligations that were stacking up. Hospital admissions, clinic visits, medications, truckloads of medical supplies and other costs were rising quickly. Our insurance through Michael's job was paying some but not all the bills. Since Amy was on dialysis, she was also eligible for Medicare. Both helped with the medical bills, but we still had all our normal obligations along with added travel expenses to the hospital. Since I could not return to work, our income had been cut in half.

Our church and the local Lions Club began fund raising to help with some of the uncovered costs. I don't know what we would have done without their help. Two gentlemen, one from our church and one from the club, spearheaded the project. Bob Allen and Floyd Crouse were God sent. Not only were our bills covered, but the worry that was removed from us was worth more than anyone could imagine. If Amy needed a medical procedure or medication that insurance refused to pay, then we could still get what she needed.

Chapter 6

The First Transplant

When Amy was about eleven months old, I sat her in the infant swing. Suddenly, she began to cry, a cry that I knew meant she was hurt. I looked down and noticed that one of her legs got caught under her. Quickly, I picked her up and repositioned her. Most children would have just stopped crying and enjoyed swinging, but Amy's medical history wasn't like most children. She kept crying and crying. I examined her but couldn't find anything wrong even though she acted like her leg was really hurting. We took her to our local hospital emergency room.

Once there, a doctor ordered an x-ray. No injuries could be found, and she was sent home. All night Amy cried; something was wrong! The next morning, I called Dr. Andreoli. She asked us to bring her to Riley.

Dr. Andreoli had Amy's leg x-rayed again. This time, two fractures could be seen with one just below her knee and the other one just above her ankle. I was really upset feeling as if it was my fault. Ordinarily a child would not have obtained a fracture this way, but Amy was in kidney failure causing brittle bones.

Amy's entire leg and foot was placed in a cast. Almost immediately, she seemed to feel better. The doctor said it would probably take a long time for her bone to heal because of the kidney failure and oxalosis. Thankfully, she was out of the cast in just six weeks. Her leg was healed!

As Amy's first birthday approached, her weight was about thirteen pounds. She could still wear newborn size diapers and clothing. The medical team discussed with us the probability of sending Amy to the University of Minnesota Hospital in Minneapolis for a transplant consultation. There, the surgeons had been performing transplants on children who weighed thirteen pounds with some success, even with oxalosis patients.

Amy was doing well considering her medical condition, but she was delayed. She couldn't sit up by herself. Her gross and fine motor skills were behind other children her age even though she was very alert mentally. She played with toys and interacted with people by cooing when spoken to and had begun to say several words. "Mama" was her first word! The delays were expected. Children in kidney failure experience physical and mental delays. I prayed constantly asking God to please protect her little brain and to let it develop normally.

In April, Michael and I flew with Amy to Minneapolis and were taken by airport shuttle to the hospital. We checked into a local hotel just blocks from the medical center which was paid for by Amy's fund. Once more, the people of Columbus made sure that Amy and her family were taken care of, and we were extremely grateful for their generosity.

Amy was admitted to the center for a multitude of tests. Since this was a medical university, Amy was seen and examined by many doctors. It was a very confusing time. One doctor would tell us one thing while the next doctor would tell us something different.

Amy's doctor told us she was sending Amy there to be under the care of Dr. Mauer. He was the physician Dr. Andreoli had trained under while at the university. Three days after Amy's admission, we had yet to meet him and were starting to wonder if he actually existed! Whenever we mentioned his name, everyone seemed to know him and remarked that he was the best doctor for Amy.

Finally, and very informally, Dr. Mauer met with the three of us in a small waiting lounge. He discussed the disease, the research he and the university were conducting and the patients with the disease who had received kidney transplants, the success and failure rates. There were three other girls, slightly older than Amy, who had received kidney transplants. Two were doing really well while the third probably would need a second transplant soon.

We received a lot of information, but the thing I would remember and hold closest to my heart was his apparent care for his young patients. There would be many members of the medical staff involved in the care of our baby. The most important thing we could do would be to determine who best we could work with and trust. He didn't know it, but it was at that moment he was chosen for that position for our baby.

During our stay, Michael and I both underwent blood tests to determine if Amy could receive one of our kidneys. Patients with oxalosis needed to receive a living related donor kidney rather than a cadaver kidney. Cadaver kidneys would sometimes take time to start working after transplantation whereas a living related donor kidney would work immediately. If a person with oxalosis had problems with the donor kidney starting, then damage to the kidney could occur before the new kidney ever kicked into action due to crystals accumulating.

We wanted the best for Amy. Because of the problems with cadaver kidneys, she would receive one of our kidneys if one of us was a good match.

The test results showed that both of us were a match with Amy. Michael was the typical match of a parent with a child; I was an even closer match. One doctor explained to us that in looking at our tissue match, it appeared Amy and I were sisters due to sharing more genes than most mothers and daughters. The only way this could be was if Michael and I shared some genes and for Amy to inherit from him the ones each of us shared. It was amazing. Even the doctor explaining the results was amazed!

The transplant was scheduled for late June, tentatively with myself as the donor. We returned home to await the exact date. Michael returned to work in order for us to keep our medical insurance and to eat! I resumed taking care of Amy and her medical needs. Bob Allen and Floyd Crouse got busy planning fund raisers.

As the date became closer, we learned that Michael would not be paid for the time off during the transplant unless donating his kidney. I also was worried about Amy's care during the time I would be hospitalized and out of commission if having the surgery. We spoke with her doctors, and they concluded it would not be a problem if Michael donated. He was as close a tissue match to her as any parent. Dr. Mauer also pointed out that should the transplant fail, as was the case of many first transplants with oxalate patients, then we would have my kidney as a backup, a closer match. That settled the matter, and Michael then had to undergo many medical tests to determine his overall health and the condition of his kidneys. He passed them all with flying colors!

Late June, we flew back to Minneapolis in preparation for the transplant. The surgery date was June 26. Amy and Michael underwent even more tests. A couple of days before the surgery, Bob Allen and one of my friends, Genora Pumphrey, arrived to be with me. It was a very scary but exciting time. We had great hopes and prayers that things would go well.

Amy even had a roommate, Stacie, who also was undergoing tests for a kidney transplant. Like Amy, she was 15 months old and was to receive her dad's kidney. Since we were undergoing the same trials, her parents and Michael and I were able to encourage and be sympathetic to each other.

Two days before the surgery, one of the surgical team doctors came in to examine Amy. She took one look at him and coughed. Concerned, he listened to her chest and back and asked about the cough. It was just a cough, I thought. She does cough occasionally even though she hadn't been coughing. He ordered a chest x-ray. It was negative, but Amy continued to cough. The doctors all went into conference together. Shortly afterwards, we received the bad news. The transplant was postponed! Due to all the immune suppressant drugs she would receive after the transplant, she could become very ill if harboring an illness. No chances could be taken! Surgery was scheduled for a week later to give them time to observe her.

We were very upset but did not want to take any chances with Amy's health. We would just wait. Bob and Genora had to return home. Bob would return in a week, but Genora would not be able to get away from her job.

Amy's cough cleared up. No diagnosis was ever made. We stayed at a local hotel that week. The doctors didn't want Amy traveling back home. Staying there, they were better able to monitor her health.

A week later, July 10, the transplant was performed. Due to jobs and other responsibilities, no one from either of our families could come for the surgery. Bob arrived. Dennis Deppa, the Church of Christ minister in nearby St. Louis Park, came to sit with me. Dennis had been visiting, praying with and encouraging us ever since our arrival in Minnesota.

The surgery took hours. Someone would come and update us on the progress. Finally, the chief transplant surgeon came out and announced the surgery was complete. Both Michael and Amy were doing well! The kidney was already functioning in Amy. He said the kidney was large, but he could get it in and close Amy up. Her abdomen was as tight as a drum, but the kidney would shrink some. I must have looked sad because he told me to smile, the worst was over. For some reason, I felt the worst was yet to come and burst into tears.

Michael returned to his room first. I went to see him, but he was very much out of it. The nurse told me he was doing well; they would take care of him and for me to concentrate on the baby. Bob Allen said he would stay with Michael and get me if needed.

Amy was finally brought back to her room on the Transplant Unit. She looked terrible! With so many wires and tubing coming from her, it was worse than when she first became ill and in intensive care at two months of age.

Her little roommate, Stacie, didn't look any better. She had her transplant earlier in the day. Both girls had their own private bedside nurse. There was so much equipment in the room that there was hardly any place to stand, let along sit down. I finally found a spot beside Amy's crib, and there I stayed. I wanted to know everything that was being done to her, and the nurse was willing to explain.

Amy was receiving so many medications including something developed by the chief transplant surgeon. This medication was supposed to help prevent rejection of the kidney. Many patients developed allergies and other complications to the drug. Amy was being monitored very carefully while seemingly not developing any negative reactions to it.

It was obvious the kidney was performing well. Urine was accumulating in her catheter bag; her kidney function tests were at the correct levels. Stacie was also doing just as well. Both girls, after a few days, were sitting up in bed, alert and interested in what was going on around them. The nurse explained they felt better than they had in a long time; they now had perfectly functioning kidneys!

Michael and Stacie's dad felt somewhat different. They had both undergone major surgery, and their bodies were adjusting to having only one kidney. We were all assured that both men would start feeling better and soon not even realize a kidney was missing.

Within a week of Amy's surgery, we started seeing signs of something not being right. Stacie's kidney function tests had leveled off; Amy's had started to climb. Her creatinine level had been a perfect 0.5, but each day it rose a little first to 0.6, then 0.7, then 0.8. Every day as the lab results were posted, my heart would drop a little further in my chest. The kidney was being damaged as the creatinine level increased!

A biopsy of her kidney was scheduled and done. Was it rejection or had the disease already started destroying her dad's kidney? We received the horrible news that the kidney was drawing oxalate crystals out of her body just as a sponge would soak up water. As this was happening, the kidney was very quickly being destroyed.

One of her doctors took me to the lab, placed one of the slides holding Amy's kidney tissue under the microscope and allowed me to see what was happening. Looking through the lens, I peered at what looked like tiny little crystals-sort of like the crystals I had seen in my dream when I was pregnant with Amy. These, the doctor explained, were what was in Amy's body and what her kidney was trying to get rid of.

I didn't know what to think. How could this be happening? My dream had become a nightmare, and we were caught up in it. I returned to Amy's room where Michael was sitting with her and tried to relay what I had seen, what was going on inside of Amy.

On the other side of the room, Stacie's parents were discussing her pending discharge with the nurse. She was doing well. Her kidney function was wonderful, and they were taking her home the next day. Some of their family had arrived from out of town, and now the parents were going out for the evening to celebrate at a bar.

I reached up and pulled the privacy drape separating the two sides of the room. Tears poured down my face as I hung my head and cried. Oh Jesus, why? I'm happy Stacie is doing well, but what about our baby? We are Christians and pray constantly. Amy is doing horrible. It seemed so ironic. Where are you, Lord? I can't seem to find you, but it seems Satan has found us. He is here in this room, mocking us.

Stacie and her parents went home. Over the next few days, Amy's creatinine continued to rise. The doctors decided nothing more could be done at this point, and Amy was discharged. We were to take her back home, under the care of her nephrologists.

Chapter 7

Return to the Hospital

Back home in Indiana, not much seemed to change initially. We didn't have to do dialysis, at least not yet, but every day that Amy's kidney function was below normal was a day that damage was still occurring to her little body.

After about a week, Amy began to vomit. At first, it appeared to be bile and then quickly changed to thick, dark vomit. I called her doctor. Without hesitation, she stressed we report to the hospital immediately so she could personally see Amy.

The doctor examined and admitted her believing she had a bowel obstruction. Amy was given a nasogastric tube hooked up to suction. This was a catheter placed up her nose and into her stomach to drain the contents that were backing up from her bowel into her stomach. We had arrived at the hospital on a Friday; thus, nothing was accomplished over the weekend except for the draining of her stomach.

It was later the following week when the doctor actually had evidence of a bowel obstruction. She conferred with Minnesota, and it was decided Amy should return to the medical center there for treatment and probably surgery. Amy and I were put on a commercial flight back. It was not a nonstop flight which presented more challenges. I was given large syringes and capped containers for use on the flight. Since Amy could not be hooked up to suction to drain her stomach, I would need to manually drain her using the syringes. I then could place the contents into the container and dispose of it during the flight. This would prevent Amy from vomiting throughout the plane trip.

When we knew we were headed to the airport, Michael called our minister. As we were standing at the gate waiting to board, we saw several men running toward us. It was Bob Allen and his friends. They had raced to the airport to pray with us before our departure. What Godly men our Jesus had brought into our lives!

Amy did not seem to be in any drastic pain with the tube, but she was very lethargic and looked very ill. I was very anxious to get her back to Minnesota. We had spent far too long sitting in the hospital in Indiana, just waiting! I was afraid of permanent damage to Amy's intestines, even gangrene.

About 20 minutes from landing somewhere to catch another flight to Minneapolis, the pilot announced we would be late. People catching the connecting flight would miss it and would have to remain there until possibly the next day. No, my brain screamed. Amy had to be on that flight! I called the flight attendant explaining Amy was due in Minneapolis that afternoon for surgery. When seeing the medical equipment and how ill Amy looked, she said she would speak to the captain. It seemed forever before she returned, but with good news. The pilot had spoken to the control tower, and they were delaying the takeoff of the connecting flight. The plane would remain on the runway until Amy and I were on board. Thank God! I knew Amy could not wait another day. Once landing, we were met by personnel who escorted us to the waiting flight. It made things so much easier, and I was so appreciative.

Michael made arrangements at home to drive to Minneapolis. It would take 18 hours to get there; so, he wouldn't be there for the surgery.

As soon as Amy was admitted, she was taken to surgery. After several hours, the surgeon came out to talk. Amy had done well. Scar tissue had caused the bowel to twist, creating the obstruction. She had been worried about all the elapsed time, but the bowel had quickly pinked back up after clipping the scar tissue loose. It was a wonderful sign, and she felt Amy would do well.

Michael arrived the next day. If Amy recovered soon, we could probably take her back home in a week to ten days. Within hours, it became obvious Amy would not be returning home any time soon. The next nine weeks proved to be worse than anything we had been through or could ever imagine!

She was ill with something other than post bowel obstruction surgery. We had to make some very difficult decisions. In the meantime, Michael had to return to work. He had already taken off so much time. We could not lose the income or the medical insurance.

Amy's temperature began to spike, sometimes as high as 105 degrees. She developed a red rash all over her body. The doctors ordered blood cultures and many other tests. What was causing Amy to be so ill? During the next few days, there were all kinds of diagnoses.

I was told she had pneumonia, a urinary tract infection, a nasal fungus and a bacteria growing in her Hickman site where a catheter went directly into her heart for blood draws. She had a constant temperature of no lower than 101 which would then spike to 105 every six hours. As her temperature rose, she would begin to shake all over and turn blue. The nurses gave her Tylenol every four hours around the clock. She was placed on a cooling blanket while no longer alert and unable to interact.

Sitting in a transplant unit and listening to nurses, doctors, and other patients and their families, a person hears all kinds of stories. I began to think Amy had contracted Cytomegalovirus or CMV as it was called. This virus would attack transplant patients with such a vengeance. The symptoms seem to fit. I asked the doctors, but they just seemed to dismiss the idea. The blood cultures hadn't come back yet, and there was no way to diagnose CMV without positive blood cultures.

Amy then developed another sign. She was losing platelets. The medical staff started giving her blood and platelet transfusions. She was so sick; I didn't think she could possibly live through it. I prayed continually and stayed by her side morning and night. I asked God to protect her brain from all the assaults so she would not be brain damaged and to give me the wisdom in making the right decisions.

I continued to receive negative reports. She developed meningitis and pulmonary edema. I was on the phone constantly, updating Michael on her condition. He wanted to return, but all he could have done was sit by her bed and watch her suffer. I convinced him to remain at home in order to keep the medical insurance we so badly needed for Amy.

I continued asking the doctors about CMV, but they refused to diagnose that until the cultures returned. There was a medication for CMV that was given to transplant patients once a week, and I inquired about Amy receiving it. It costs thousands of dollars per dose and could not be given without a diagnosis. I was afraid Amy would die before we could get the diagnosis and was extremely frustrated with a system that was denying Amy what I felt sure she needed.

Her platelets kept falling, and she kept needing transfusions. One of the surgeons decided her transplanted kidney was destroying her platelets. The surgeon practically demanded to take Amy to surgery to remove her kidney. I refused. Then she became hateful saying, "You are going to kill Amy!"

I replied, "The CMV is causing the platelet problem."

"You don't know that as a fact."

Looking her right in the eye, "If you take my daughter to surgery in her present condition, then Amy will die."

The surgeon stomped her foot, spun around and left the room, obviously very angry.

It just happened that this conversation was witnessed by a hospital social worker, Linda, who had come in the room to visit and had been sitting in a corner. She asked if the doctor was always that hateful. I shared her attitude changed when I refused the surgery. Linda was very concerned and wanted me to bring charges to the hospital ethics board. I didn't have the strength. All of it was going to Amy, and all I wanted was to have Amy well and healthy. I had to make decisions for Amy based on what I felt in my heart. Linda, however, made a complaint herself about the doctor. The next time I saw the doctor, she was cordial and made no demands about the surgery.

One night, I gave up as I stood beside Amy's crib while the fever raged. I could no longer bear to watch her suffer. I asked God to either heal or take her to keep her from suffering. I lay down on the cot and felt so empty inside and so sad at the same time. I didn't know when it would be, but at some point I would have to call Michael and let him know she was gone.

I was awakened sometime toward morning by a nurse talking to Amy. Amy's temperature was the lowest it had been-100 degrees. I got up from the cot and went to the crib. Amy was awake, and she was looking at us. From that moment on, Amy steadily began to improve despite being so weak and losing everything she had ever learned. She could not even hold her head up, could no longer talk, not even say mama. I picked her up and cuddled her. It seemed she still knew who I was.

Amy shook terribly and didn't have any control over her little hands and fingers. As I watched her struggle to reach and grasp her pacifier, I worried about brain damage. But she would look up at me, and I could still see in her eyes that the Amy I knew was still there.

We helped her regain strength in her neck and back. About the time she started to get better, we received the lab report of her blood cultures for CMV. They were positive! The doctors started giving her the medication once a week by IV.

Of course, I wondered how much of her suffering could have been avoided! I could have become very bitter dwelling on this, but something seemed to say that it didn't matter. Amy got well, not because of the medication she was given, but because I had surrendered her to God.

I bought Amy a toy plastic bottle with a large opening and some poker chips. These bright colored chips stimulated her to pick them up and place them in the bottle. It started out as a very difficult game due to the loss of her fine motor muscle control, but it wasn't long before she was actually picking up the one she wanted and placing it in the bottle.

As the weeks went by, Amy continued to improve physically, mentally and socially. She started babbling again and surprised me one day by saying "mama" while looking at me. Tears streamed down my face. My baby was back, and she knew who I was!

Chapter 8

The Move

The doctors decided to put her back on dialysis and on hemodialysis. Her kidney function was still fair, but the oxalate crystals were continuing to accumulate in her body. Hemodialysis would help pull the crystals from her blood better than peritoneal dialysis. She was scheduled for dialysis three times a week for four to six hours.

A meeting was scheduled with the doctors. Michael, myself and the social workers met to discuss Amy's future. We met while Amy was in dialysis. It was a very difficult session. I knew Amy was such a fighter and wanted to live. There was still so much life in her yet to be lived.

We discussed how Amy was doing since surviving what many other patients had not. She actually was doing really well. The last child that suffered CMV and other infections as Amy had been left blind and brain damaged to the degree that she was like an infant even though she was eight years old. The child would require total care for the rest of her life.

There was also a little three-year-old oxalate patient, Lucy, whose transplant had occurred about two years prior to Amy's. She, like Amy, had oxalate reoccurrence in her transplanted kidney almost from the start. Over the next two years, she had barely grown. There was minimal kidney function, and the crystals had gathered in her body causing many bone fractures. At the time of our meeting, the little girl was back on dialysis with a complete body cast due to her many fractures.

We discussed the possibility of another transplant. If I were to donate my kidney, I would have a one in 1000 chance of not surviving like all living related donors. My chances of dying during surgery were greater than the chances of another kidney transplant being successful for Amy.

In other words, it sounded as if they really doubted another transplant would ever succeed for Amy. I could not just do nothing for Amy, not when she had pulled through so much and continued to improve every day. The meeting was long and very exhausting, not only for us but also for the doctors. It was very evident that they cared deeply about their patients. We eventually reached an agreement. Amy would be placed on a waiting list for a cadaver kidney. If a kidney could not be found in six months, she would receive mine. I was concerned because a cadaver kidney might not work even if finding a match. At the same time, we had the approval for another transplant. We would just have to trust God.

It was late September 1984; Amy and I were stuck in Minneapolis. Michael was back in Indiana working and flying up when possible. This was depleting her fund money. We made the decision that we all needed to live in Minnesota. The company Michael worked for could transfer him to the Minneapolis area. There would be no pay increase. With living expenses higher in Minneapolis and rent alone substantially higher, we wondered how we could possibly meet our budget.

After discussions with Bob Allen and Floyd Crouse, we all determined that the remaining fund raiser monies would pay our rent during the six months before and for several months after the surgery. Each month there, Bob would send us a check for the rent. We could then manage to live on

Michael's pay check. We were so grateful for the people in and around Columbus, Indiana. They had provided the money so desperately needed for Amy and our family, and now we could be together.

In early October, Amy and I flew home to Indiana. People from our church helped me pack, and Michael loaded the rented truck. Amy and I flew back to Minneapolis to the house we had rented. Dennis Deppa, pastor of St. Louis Park Church of Christ, met us at the airport and took us to the house. It was empty. Michael would follow in a few days with all our belongings. Dennis and his wife, Delores, offered to let us stay at their house, but I felt Amy and I needed to be in our own home. I made a pallet on the floor, and that's where we slept. Amy's hospital stays had taught me to sleep wherever I could find a place to lie down.

The next day, Amy and I started our three times a week 20 mile trek from that home to the University of Minnesota Medical Center for treatments. She had occupational, physical and speech therapy in the morning and dialysis in the afternoon. Since I no longer had to deal with peritoneal dialysis and the additional feeding problems they caused, I had the time to just play with Amy. I talked to her constantly and worked with her to build up her muscles and strengthen them for her second transplant.

Amy's feedings were no longer a struggle. While in the hospital, the doctors decided Amy would be tube fed. Every night, I would pass a nasogastric tube up Amy's nose and down her esophagus into her stomach. I would then attach the tube to a bag of feeding. All night, a pump would slowly pump formula into her stomach. I could have left the tube in all day and just clamped it off, but I really wanted Amy to appear as normal as possible. Consequently, I would pull out the tube every morning and reinsert it at night. If Amy had objected, I would have left it in. She would help me put the tube down by sucking on her pacifier and swallowing as I passed the tube beyond her throat and into her stomach. In the morning, she would hold very still as I removed it. The procedure would throw her into a fit of sneezing, and she would squeal with delight and laugh when the sneezing stopped.

We managed to settle into a routine living in Minnesota. Michael would help care for Amy, play and work with her on therapy exercises when home. This gave me a little time for household duties. If I was not taking a shower or if Amy was in dialysis, then I was holding her. I was so afraid of her choking at night vomiting on her feeding that I even let her sleep with us. She was most comfortable lying on my chest which she did for months. As the doctors figured out her feeding and medications, vomiting at night became fairly rare.

One day, we received the call we had been waiting for. There was a kidney available! We were unsure about using a cadaver kidney but would not turn one down. I called Michael at work to meet us at the hospital and then packed Amy's stuff up. It had been a non-dialysis day and a good one for Amy; so, we had been home just spending time together. On the drive to the hospital, I prayed that this would be a perfect kidney. I had been told nothing about the donor but prayed for the family who was making this donation.

When I got to the hospital and reached in the car seat to pick Amy up, I sensed something was wrong. She felt so warm. We were to meet one of the doctors, Dr. Chavers, on the dialysis unit who was to examine Amy before sending us to the transplant unit. She took one look at Amy and asked why she was so red. I thought she had a temperature. Sure enough, a thermometer indicated a temperature of 102. She had been fine 30 minutes prior! How could she have a 102 temp now?

Dr. Chavers ordered blood cultures, urine cultures and a chest x-ray. She checked her ears and throat with no signs of infection. The chest x-ray was negative, no sign of pneumonia. Stripped down and sitting on an exam table, her temperature remained up. It would be at least 24 hours before we received the results of the urine and blood cultures. Her urine was clear, no visible signs of infection. Dr. Chavers doubted that she had sepsis. What was wrong with her? Amy did not appear ill except for being flushed.

Dr. Chavers turned her attention from Amy to me. She didn't know what was wrong, but she could not allow the transplant. It would be too risky. I understood, but I couldn't understand how or why Amy had developed a fever. The doctor asked if I was comfortable taking Amy home or if I preferred admitting her for the night. I elected to watch her closely at home.

Driving back home, Amy acted normal. She babbled and played. After arriving home, I found her temperature to be normal. Picking her up, I told her that she obviously didn't want that kidney. She squealed and wrapped her little arms around my neck squeezing tightly.

Later in the week, during dialysis, we met the husband of the patient who received the kidney. The woman was not doing well; the kidney had not starting working. I felt really bad for the woman. Once again, I felt like God was listening to our prayers to protect Amy.

I worried constantly about our decisions. Were we doing the right things? Amy had suffered so much after her first transplant. Now, she seemed happy, smiling and enjoying life. I really did not want to put Amy through any more medical procedures only delaying a certain death, if in the end she was going to die anyway. There were things far worse than death; I had seen them! As much as it pained me at the thought of being without her, I preferred Amy to be in the arms of Jesus then to undergo any more suffering. I begged God to tell me if Amy was going to live, if not, to let me know so we could let her go. Another decision could not be made unless He answered this question!

One evening, we received another call about a child's donated kidney. The doctors preferred Amy receive an adult kidney because of the fluids required after the surgery. They wanted to push lots of fluid through the kidney after the transplant in hopes of washing out any crystals before they accumulated. A child's kidney might not be able to handle all the fluid. I was home alone with Amy; Michael was at work; I couldn't make a decision. It was a really good kidney, one they felt would work right away. The caller said he would call one of Amy's nephrologists and discuss it. Someone would call back. I called Michael. He too was torn by the decision and wasn't sure what to decide.

I paced the floor with Amy in my arms while crying and praying, not wanting to put her through another surgery unless it was the best decision. What was the best decision?

The phone rang, and it was one of Amy's kidney doctors. She wasn't sure what to do either. We talked and finally decided that Dr. Mauer knew about oxalosis and kidney transplants better than anyone. He also knew Amy. We would let him make the decision. I hung up and prayed like crazy. Please let Dr. Mauer know what to decide.

A little while later, the phone rang. It was Dr. Mauer. He discussed the pros and cons of using the kidney and felt we should turn the kidney down. I agreed with the decision. He would let the transplant coordinator know. I didn't know whether to be relieved or cry in disappointment. So, I prayed.

"Lord, I cannot do this any longer. You are going to have to decide if Amy should have another transplant, and you are going to have to let me know if Amy is to live or not. I cannot go on like this."

I had never felt so desperate in all my life. Suddenly, I heard a voice, "Read John 4:10."

I knew there was a God, seeing him at work numerous times, but I had never heard his voice and certainly didn't know where anything was in the Bible. For years, I hadn't read it because I found it difficult to understand.

I placed Amy on a blanket on the floor and went in search of my Bible. I found John in the New Testament, opened it to John 4:10 and read "If you only knew what a wonderful gift God had for you and who I <u>am, y</u>ou would ask me for some <u>living</u> water."

I stared at the words. The words "amy" and "living" seemed to jump out. There it was in Jesus' own words. Right there were the words I needed. It would be years before I completely understood this verse.

Amy was going to live, and, because God had said so, she would have a good life! I would remember this moment for the rest of my life, and I would have a wonderful story to tell Amy of how God had responded to her mother's desperate plea for an answer.

After hearing our Lord's voice, I now had hope that things would change. But, the thing that really needed to change was me. I had to accept the fact that Amy was going to be healed even if it wasn't the way I wanted, an instant miracle. If instead it came through a kidney transplant, then it would work out perfectly because God had promised she would live. I just had to accept and trust.

Chapter 9

Christmas with Jimmy

So life continued. Amy and I continued our three times a week trek to the center for therapy and dialysis. Dialysis lasted four to six hours, and I would stay with Amy the entire session. Things could turn bad suddenly, and I felt a need to be there in case it did. While Amy slept, my attention would be captured by the patients and their families.

One patient that caught my attention was a little boy who appeared to be about Amy's age. He would arrive with a staff member shortly after Amy's dialysis treatment started and would be handed over to a dialysis nurse. She would return after the treatment to retrieve him. He usually slept through the treatment too.

One day, he was awake and sitting up in the crib. I was looking at him wondering about his parents. I had never seen them. Suddenly, I must have caught his eye because he turned his head and stared at me for several minutes from across the room. Where is your mother, I wondered to myself? How could a mother just send her baby to something like dialysis all by himself? I wanted to know his story and asked one of the dialysis nurses.

Jimmy was from another state quite far away. He had been born to a mother who was struggling with several problems. Since he was not healthy at birth, his mother could not cope with all the responsibilities. For whatever reason, she would not give permission for Jimmy to receive the medical care he needed. His single father stepped in, married the mother so he could obtain custody and signed for Jimmy's medical treatment. The University of Minnesota was the closest facility with the medical knowledge that could care for Jimmy. Jimmy was now 28 months old and had never been out of the hospital. His father would make the long trip when he could. Often, Jimmy had no one except the medical staff, and they went home every day to their own families.

When hearing this story, I was so saddened by it. What if I had to leave Amy somewhere else where I couldn't be there for the medical care needed? I didn't think I could bear such a situation.

As Christmas approached, I kept thinking of Jimmy. My little family was so far away from everyone else we knew and loved, but at least we had each other. Finally, I knew what I had to do. While Amy was in dialysis getting treated, I went to see the hospital social worker, Ella. We had known her now for months, and I knew she was a caring, compassionate woman.

When expressing I wanted to take Jimmy home to spend Christmas with us, she thought it would be wonderful, but not possible. We would have to get permission from Jimmy's father, his legal guardian. Jimmy's father loved him very much and would not let go of him. Many of the staff nurses had tried to take Jimmy home with them, but his father always refused permission. Ella was not sure exactly why but felt he was perhaps very scared of losing his son. I begged her to at least ask.

The following week after Amy was settled on the dialysis unit, I searched out Ella who had me sit down when entering her office. She had spoken with Jimmy's father and was completely blown away. He would let Jimmy spend Christmas Eve night at our house. I was overjoyed. It would be Jimmy's first trip out of the hospital, and my family would get to be a part of it!

Michael, Amy and I picked Jimmy up from the hospital early Christmas Eve. Amy was excited; another child was coming to play with her! We weren't sure how Jimmy felt. He couldn't talk, couldn't walk, and it was difficult to read any emotion on his face even though his eyes were huge as we placed him in our car.

Our first bit of excitement was something Amy enjoyed but Jimmy had never experienced, a trip to the toy store. We put him in a cart just as we did Amy and pushed them both up and down the aisles. Amy babbled and pointed at the pretty colors on the packages. She would say the few words she could, laugh, throw her head back and look at the shelves piled high with toys.

Jimmy's eyes would just seem to get bigger as we pushed them down the aisles. We showed him toys but couldn't tell if he preferred one over the other. Finally, we picked some out so he could have presents to open Christmas morning.

That evening, we took both children to a candlelight service at church. People would come up to meet Jimmy and shake his little hand. He would just stare at them, and I so wished I could read his mind.

In the morning, Amy woke me up patting my face and bouncing up and down between Michael and me. I raised up to look at Jimmy. He was awake in the crib peering at us between the bars. Amy continued to bounce and sing, pulling on her daddy to wake him up too. He rolled over, picked her up, tossed her up in the air and caught her as she came down while they both laughed. There we were kissing and loving on each other on this special Christmas morning. Jimmy sat and watched us. Michael climbed out of bed, picked him up and deposited him between us and close to Amy. She laughed, grabbed his fat little cheek and squeezed it. He didn't seem to mind.

We stayed that way for some time, the four of us hugging, kissing while Michael and I tickled their fat little tummies. I never saw Jimmy smile, and I wondered if his face muscles knew how. I just hoped that maybe his heart was smiling because mine was for the first time in months.

After Christmas was over and we had returned Jimmy to the hospital, I could not get my mind off the fact that he actually had to live there and could not go home. I approached Ella once more. Michael and I wanted to become Jimmy's foster parents. Ella explained it would take months, even if the father felt it would be better. We would have to become licensed by the state first. She would check into the requirements.

We were never able to accomplish this arrangement. Jimmy received a kidney transplant. During the surgery, due to complications in Jimmy's abnormal anatomy, the surgeon accidentally and unknowingly cut Jimmy's bowel. He became very ill and passed away within days of the surgery. However, Jimmy left me with the desire in my heart to foster other children which remained and became a reality 16 years later!

Chapter 10

The Second Transplant

Amy's transplant, using my kidney, was scheduled for March 07, 1985. During the previous six months, we had only received two calls about an available cadaver kidney. Michael and I received an opportunity to speak with a doctor that handled the incoming calls regarding available donated organs. Amy had antibodies against only eight percent of the average population which ordinarily was quite the positive. Other kidneys had come in; however, Amy always had antibodies against them. It was very unusual since her antibody level was so low. The doctor couldn't explain it, but Michael and I could understand it. Amy was destined to receive my kidney!

We awakened the morning of March 7 to the most snow I had ever seen in my life. Minneapolis had a blizzard during the night. The roads were impassable. We couldn't find the car, let alone get it on the road, and we didn't know how we were going to get Amy to the hospital. Fortunately, Minnesota was accustomed to snow and knew how to handle it. Within hours, the roads were clear enough to drive four-wheel vehicles on them. Pastor Dennis sent someone to pick us up and deliver the three of us to the hospital.

Amy was admitted to the Transplant Unit. I didn't have to report to my Admitting Unit until the next morning. I slept in Amy's room while Michael spent the night in the waiting room.

The following morning, I reported to my unit where I was informed I could stay with Amy in her room until needed. Michael and I hung out in Amy's room between her many tests.

Michael was stranded at the hospital during the night because of the storm. Someone from social services located a place for him to shower and change clothing. He was able to eat breakfast in the hospital cafeteria. I decided to spend the time with Amy and wait until later to go to my room for a shower. Due to the surgery scheduled for the next day, I could not eat.

At 11:30, Amy's nurse told me I was needed on my unit immediately. I went to the unit and was met by my nurse as well as a transport person who would be taking me to the Gynecology Clinic. They had scheduled a 12:00 appointment for a pelvic exam.

I panicked since not showering for two days and due to not understanding why a pelvic exam had been ordered. I was donating my kidney to Amy, not my uterus! The nurse couldn't explain, but I had to have the exam in order to have the kidney surgery. I refused to go until showering and took the fastest one ever with two people standing at the door rushing me every two minutes. I had never been to a doctor in my life without first taking a shower, and I wasn't about to start now. I skipped the makeup and combed my hair as we practically ran through tunnels to a neighboring building. We arrived just as my appointment time came up on the clinic clock.

In the exam room, I questioned the need for the exam and found out it was necessary to be sure I wasn't pregnant. I could have told them that!

The next morning, a nurse arrived and gave me the pre-op medications. I was then taken to a holding area to Amy. Someone placed her on my gurney, and we were able to cuddle for a while. Then, we were separated and headed toward adjoining surgery rooms. Just as we went through the door, the electricity went off. The generators kicked on, turning on emergency lights. I wondered if this was some terrible sign. No one seemed to know why. I felt groggy from the pre-op meds and couldn't think straight. Someone announced that the storm had knocked out the electricity. Surgeries were canceled until further notice. I was pushed back to the holding area. There, we were informed the surgeries would resume when the electricity had been restored. Due to the pre-op medicine I had been given, I slept until we were put back on the schedule.

The next thing I knew, I was in surgery. The anesthesiologist was telling me to count backwards from 100. I looked at the clock on the wall. It was 2:02 p.m. I got to 97 and was fast asleep. I was unaware of it, but surgery had begun.

When I awakened, I was in terrible pain. A doctor was bending over me and telling me to wake up. I wanted to tell him I was awake and to leave me alone! When realizing where I was and why, I had to know about Amy. I asked if her kidney was working and he said "so far." What did that mean? Were they expecting it to quit working? I complained of the pain, and the nurse gave me something for it right then. I fell back to sleep.

When awakening, I was being pushed on a gurney back into my room. Michael was there, and I asked why he wasn't with Amy. He had come to check on me. Amy was doing well. I insisted that he stay with her.

The entire night, I suffered from severe hiccoughs. I kept waking up in horrible pain. A nurse would put medicine in my IV line, and I would fall asleep only to wake back up to repeat the cycle. As the sun rose, a couple of nurses requested I stand up so they could weigh me. At first, I thought I was dreaming. Stand up? I couldn't even get out of the fetal position! They began pulling on me, stood me up and then had me step on the scales. The next thing I knew, the male nurse had me in his arms and was placing me back in the bed. I passed out on them!

I continued to hiccough. It felt like someone had placed a hot poker in my side and was twisting it. The nurses kept shooting me up with Thorazine, a drug to stop the hiccoughs. The doctors were concerned about the cause of the hiccoughs and ordered a portable x-ray of my abdomen. Thank God it was portable! I never would have made it to the x-ray department without a repeat of the morning passing out episode.

The x-ray came back negative. Throughout the day, which was Friday, I would wake up long enough to ask about Amy only to hiccough, moan and receive more Thorazine. Late in the day, my mind cleared enough that I told a nurse that Demerol caused Amy to have hiccoughs. I am not sure why because my mind was too drugged to think clearly. The nurse took that information to my doctor. The Demerol for my pain was discontinued, and the hiccoughs stopped. Apparently, Amy and I shared the same drug idiosyncrasy to Demerol.

Saturday morning, I awakened more alert since I was no longer receiving Demerol or Thorazine. I wanted to see Amy! Michael went and received permission for me to leave the unit. I wanted to walk to the elevator; I needed to get back on my feet to care for Amy. The nurse told Michael to follow with a wheelchair. I made it to the elevator but then had to sit down.

Michael wheeled me to Amy's room, but I was determined to walk in to see her.

When entering the room, Amy was sitting up in her crib, playing. Her nurse was beside the bed and explained that Amy was doing wonderfully. I spoke to Amy. She looked at me, stuck her chin up and turned her head! She was mad at me. I had just let her go through surgery and had not been there afterward for the first time.

It hurt; I had just given life to her and she was mad at me! I sat down in a chair, and Michael placed her in my lap. She wouldn't look at me, wouldn't even touch me. I sat there and talked explaining where I had been and how much I loved her. She kept glancing at me out of the corners of her eyes. Suddenly, she smiled. She couldn't act mad any longer! She reached out her hand and touched mine. I hugged her, and she cuddled up. She had forgiven me for my absence the past two days. I cried. I was in so much pain physically, but I would do it again, just for this precious little girl in my arms. I would go through anything to see her healthy!

I was discharged on Tuesday and instructed not to lift anything over ten pounds. That was a problem. Amy weighed 18 pounds, and she still couldn't walk. Michael needed to go back to work and would not be available to help. While Amy was in the hospital, it wasn't much of a problem because the nurses were there to help. Once she was discharged, I would not have any help. But, I wanted her home as soon as possible!

We watched Amy's lab results closely as her blood was drawn every day. Until receiving the results, I felt like my stomach was sitting in my throat. Once posted and still normal, I could relax, at least for one more day.

Amy's new kidney was working well. The medications and the high fluid intake apparently were keeping this kidney safe. She was discharged on March 21, my 29th birthday. I didn't get to celebrate long because she developed a fever and was readmitted to the hospital with a temperature of 102 the following day. I was terrified! Was she already rejecting the kidney? She remained in the hospital until April 5 with a flu virus. I was so relieved when Amy was released!

Chapter 11

Amy is Healthy!

At home, Amy was gaining strength and making attempts to walk. We were amazed at what a difference a working kidney made. Amy had always been a happy, smiling child, but now she smiled and laughed all the time. It didn't bother us when she started to get into everything. She was over two years of age but looked about ten months old even though she seemed to understand things like a much older child. Watching her play and interact with her environment, I was convinced that no brain damage had occurred.

Life seemed good for the first time in a long time. Amy was healthy; her kidney function tests proved the kidney was working perfectly. We started checking into preschools for fall while wanting her to catch up with other children as quickly as possible.

In early June, Amy became ill again and was readmitted to the hospital due to vomiting and a fever. She wanted me in bed with her. After all she had been through, I didn't mind. I loved holding her tiny little body against mine. There had been so many medical procedures, and I knew she was afraid every time we were separated.

We were probably both snoring when the nurse awakened me. An intern was standing beside her with syringes and needles in his hand saying, "We need to draw Any's blood for labs."

Amy immediately opened her big, brown eyes. Tears filled them as she grabbed onto me. Her little body was shaking as she clutched tightly crying, "No, mama, no!"

"Let me get her completely awake first," I requested. I wouldn't want to be awakened in this manner, and I wasn't going to let them do it to Amy.

"I don't have time for this; I have to do her now," the intern practically snarled at me.

"No," I repeated. "You are not jabbing needles in her the minute she wakes up. She is terrified."

Amy was clinging to me, still shaking while crying out, "No, mama, no."

"Like I said, I don't have time this morning for this. Lay her down so I can draw her blood."

The intern was as angry as Amy was frightened. I was just as determined in my feelings to protect her from the beast as I'm sure Amy thought of him.

"No, you can wait a few minutes." I hated arguing with this man, but Amy could not speak for herself. His face turned red, and he threw a hand up. I thought he was going to hit me.

The nurse touched his arm and gently said, "You have the child next door to draw also. Go do him, then come back to Amy."

He threw the supplies down on the bedside table and angrily stomped out of the room. I was grateful for the nurse's intervention and thanked her.

I pulled Amy's stiff little body free from my shoulder. "Look, Amy. He is gone."

She turned her head and looked, the fear leaving her eyes. "Bad man gone," she said.

I felt her relax as she cuddled, and I placed her little hand in mine. After a few minutes, I would explain why we needed to let the bad man come back. We didn't have a choice.

How was I going to get her to understand he wasn't really a bad man? It was hard for me to understand at times! In order to protect Amy from some insensitivity at times of a busy staff, I found myself arguing with them now and then. I just prayed they would be professional enough to not take it out on her. It was determined that Amy had another virus, and she was soon released.

In July, an unexpected bomb dropped. I was pregnant! Michael and I had decided we would not have any more children. We could not take the chance of another child having oxalosis. My birth control had not changed. I could not figure out how this had occurred, but a visit to the doctor confirmed it.

Just like my pregnancy with Amy, morning sickness lasted from morning until night. I couldn't keep anything down and mostly stayed on the sofa beside a plastic pail while not moving except to provide care for Amy. The doctor wanted to admit me to the hospital, but I refused. There was no one to take care of Amy. We were several states away from our families, and Michael had to work.

The doctor emphasized on a Wednesday that if I was unable to keep any food or liquid down that I would be admitted to the hospital on Friday. What would we do? Even if Michael took off work, he was not that familiar with all of Amy's medications. I could not leave her! I started praying I would be able to eat and drink something. Dehydration was not good for the unborn baby either.

Searching the refrigerator, I found some popsicles and slowly began eating one. It stayed down. Over the next few hours, I sucked on a popsicle constantly. Later, I found a bag of Cracker Jacks and slowly began to munch on them. They stayed down too. By Friday, I was able to report I had eaten the whole box of popsicles and the bag of Cracker Jacks. The doctor extended my deadline until Monday to keep other food down. Gradually, my diet improved even though I still vomited several times each day throughout the pregnancy.

The doctor talked with us about having an amniocentesis to check for oxalosis in the fetus. When inquiring about the process, Dr. Mauer explained that at that time no one knew what to do with the results once obtained. Would a high level indicate the child had oxalosis or not? No one knew. If a high level was suspected of indicating oxalosis, then he asked if I would consider an abortion? I could not.

We decided against the amniocentesis. It would have been good to have the results for research, but I could not bring myself to undergo it. I would have wanted to know the results and would have driven myself crazy wondering what they meant.

In August, the three of us moved in The Potter's House. This was a home away from home for transplant patients and their families at the University of Minnesota Medical Center. It was run like a Ronald McDonald House, a place for cancer patients and their families at various hospitals throughout the United States. Michael and I were asked to be resident managers for the facility. There, we would remain for the next two years. We met many patients and their families as they came to the hospital for consultations, transplants and follow-up care and became very close to many of them. We rejoiced in their victories and cried with them in their sorrow.

In October, we placed Amy at two and a half in a preschool program for children with special needs. She was walking but not talking as well as other children her age and had eating problems because of being tube fed most of her life. Amy would drink but would refuse food because she just didn't know how to eat. We had hopes that being around other children would help.

Due to the oxalosis, there were many foods Amy would never be allowed to eat. She also could not have anything high in Vitamin C. The school was willing to work with us on the special diet as she learned to eat.

The first day of school, I was reluctant to leave her. The staff allowed me to stay and observe. They knew I was having a more difficult time letting go than Amy. It was a good thing I was there.

The teachers had taken the children into the gym. Amy slipped and fell and immediately began crying. The fall appeared to be minor, but she was sounding as if something was wrong. She kept holding her leg. I could tell by the way she cried that the leg was probably fractured. The school's physical therapist came, checked her and said she didn't think there was any major injury. Well versed in her background and cries, I decided to take her to be x-rayed as a precaution.

Once the x-ray was done, we knew for sure that Amy's leg was fractured. The break was at the site of the ankle break which had occurred when she was an infant. Her leg and foot was placed in a cast, so much for walking and an uneventful beginning to school! Amy had to wear the cast for six weeks.

It wasn't easy carrying her around with a cast on her leg while pregnant. The Potter's House had stairs everywhere. We had to take stairs to get to the main living area, stairs to get down to the kitchen area, stairs to the bedroom area and stairs to our own apartment. As I lugged Amy and her cast up and down the stairs, I felt as though I would have the baby soon even though barely six months along.

At the end of six weeks, I took Amy in to have her cast removed. Since Amy's bones were so brittle, the doctor felt the cast should remain on another four weeks. I almost cried, and he asked why it was a problem. I told him to envision being seven months pregnant, carrying Amy and a long cast up and down multiple steps. He believed keeping the cast on longer would help Amy's leg heal better. I would just have to cope with it!

When her cast was finally removed in early January, she felt so light. We both felt so much better! The evening after she had it removed, I was standing at our apartment door talking with one of the home's occupants. Amy played in the hall, stepping on and off the bottom step. Suddenly, she fell before I could catch her. She screamed in pain. As I carried her back into our apartment, she continued to cry and hold her foot. As I examined it, I couldn't see any injury but knew from previous experiences to take her to the emergency room.

There, her foot and leg were x-rayed, and she had fractured her foot. She was put back into a cast up to her knee for another six weeks. I held her and cried, feeling so guilty for allowing her to play on the step. Were her bones ever going to get strong enough to play like a normal child? She had a walking cast this time, and it didn't slow her down. She resumed walking with the cast as well as she had before without it. By mid-February, the cast was removed. For the next few weeks, I worried every time she so much as moved.

Chapter 12

A Sister is Born

I was 37 weeks pregnant on Monday, March 10 and had an appointment with my obstetrician. Ever since Amy was in casts, I felt the baby would come early. Every time I picked her up, I thought my insides were going to drop out. Climbing all the stairs did not help. But, after the doctor examined me, I was assured this baby would enter the world in three weeks.

The doctor then sent me for an ultrasound. I would have one every week until the baby was born. He wanted to watch the amount of amniotic fluid surrounding the baby; a low amount could indicate kidney failure in the baby.

I had to stay on my back during the ultrasound. As the technician ran the probe over my abdomen, I began to feel as if I was going to pass out. I wanted to sit up, but he kept saying it would only take a couple more minutes. With each second, I felt as if I was dying. His assistant, a female, stopped the technician and had me turn on my side which provided instant relief. When they restarted the ultrasound procedure, I became very ill again. They explained the baby was pressing down on my aorta, and the pressure from the ultrasound probe made it worse. This caused the blood to return slowly to my head creating the ill feelings. Whatever caused it, I didn't want to repeat this every week for the next three weeks. At the same time, I knew the doctor needed the results from the tests for the baby's sake.

The following day, Michael, Amy and I appeared on a local TV show. The show was about the Potter's House and the people who were staying there. We hoped the exposure would bring in more funding for the house. I was relieved when the show was over; I was tired and just wanted to go home!

The next morning, Michael left for work. Amy and I went to the playroom in the house. As we played together, I began to have cramps which got worse as the morning progressed. I called my doctor, the one who told me I had three weeks to go, and he said to report to the hospital if the cramps continued. I called Michael. It was noon, and he was scheduled to work until 4 p.m. I suggested he remain at work; I would call him if needed. During the afternoon, I got Amy's medicine ready for the next three days.

Michael arrived home at 4:45, and he was extremely anxious when discovering my labor pains were three minutes apart. I had spoken with a woman staying at the house about caring for Amy. Nancy had been there for months waiting for a heart transplant for her husband, and we had grown close. He had just received a new heart and now had to remain in the area for many weeks before the doctors would dismiss him to return home. Nancy was more than happy to help us out with Amy while Michael was at the hospital. With Amy and her medicine taken care of, we were off to the hospital which was only three blocks away. It was just after 6 p.m. Katie was born at 9:07 p.m.

While I was in labor, Michael insisted we pick out a boy's name. He wanted a boy! From the moment I was pregnant, I knew it would be another girl. She would also have blond hair and blue eyes. Amy had brown hair and brown eyes; so, I'm not sure how I knew this little girl would look so different. She would be Katie Rose. No matter what, we both knew there would not be any more children.

Over the next three hours, Michael kept urging me to choose a boy's name. I was not in the mood, especially when just knowing it would be a girl. As our baby was born and only halfway out-head first, Michael yelled, "It's a boy!"

I looked down in shock; there was no way to tell at that particular moment. Being in a horrible mood, I could have hit Michael. Suddenly, the baby slid out. I managed to look at Michael and say, "I told you so."

When our baby was handed to me, I could see her blond hair and beautiful blue eyes. I asked Michael if he was disappointed. His loving look at the little 5 pound 10 ounce girl in my arms was my answer. I had worried during my pregnancy if I could possibly love another child as much as Amy. As I held and nursed her the next day, there was no doubt.

Thursday was spent having tests run on Katie Rose and talking with doctors. Ella, the social worker, came to visit on Friday. While there, one of the kidney doctors came in to give me the results of the oxalosis tests. The tests indicated Katie had the disease. As he left, Michael walked in. When I told him what the doctor had said, he walked over and took her from my arms. He then carried her over to a chair and sat down. As he stared at her, he began to sob. While Amy had been ill, I had seen him very upset but had never seen him cry until that moment. I was already crying. As I looked up at Ella, I could see tears flowing down her cheeks. This precious little baby wasn't even two full days old yet, and our hearts were already breaking over her!

Later that day, another doctor came in to give us more bad news. I had been found to be Cytomegalovirus positive. This meant I had been exposed to the virus at some point. Amy had CMV, and I probably had caught it from her. Most healthy people are barely ill when contracting the virus like me; however, babies born to CMV positive mothers were very ill. Katie would need to be transferred to the infant intensive care unit.

It was more than I could hardly bear-Oxalosis and now CMV, all in one day. My doctor was discharging me, and I would have to leave Katie at the hospital. When the nurse came to take Katie to the Intensive Care Unit, we also went. As we walked into the unit, the nurse who would be caring for Katie came up to me and obviously could tell I was upset. She put an arm around me and said, "Don't you worry. I have seen a lot of CMV infected babies. Your baby does not have CMV; I don't care what the doctors say. She would be very ill at this point if she did."

I don't know who that nurse was because of never seeing her again, but I was so thankful. She had given me hope! Perhaps she really had been an angel, sent by God to encourage me. I left my baby in her care, and Michael took me home to rest. My intentions were to return at midnight to nurse her, but I was too exhausted to get out of bed. Michael called the unit requesting them to go ahead and bottle feed her.

Katie remained in the Intensive Care Unit for two days. When it became obvious she was not ill and did not have any effects from the CMV, she was transferred to the Infant Care

Unit. They could not transfer her back to the Newborn Nursery once being discharged from there due to hospital policy.

While in the Infant Care Unit, the doctors figured out the doses of medication she would need for the oxalosis. We all hoped they could ward off kidney failure at least until she was older. This approach had never been attempted, but the doctors thought it was worth trying.

Katie was discharged on Tuesday. We returned to the clinic on Thursday. I was met by one of the kidney doctors. Previous tests showed Katie had a urinary tract infection and probably contracted it when the nurses cathed her bladder for urine tests. She would have to be readmitted to the hospital for IV antibiotics. I just stood and cried. The poor doctor didn't know what to say. I think she felt almost as bad as I did. She just stood and patted me on the back.

Katie was readmitted, and an IV was started into a vein in her little head. It was March 20. The next day was my 30th birthday. For two straight years, I had sat in the hospital with an ill child on my birthday. Fortunately, Katie's urinary tract infection was found to be susceptible to an oral antibiotic. She was discharged on March 22. I would give her the antibiotic at home along with the medications for the oxalosis.

Several days after Katie came home, I was holding her and feeling very depressed. I could not stand the thought of her going through what Amy had suffered. She was beautiful. I questioned God. Even though I believed He would never give us more than we could bear, I felt He had done exactly that. How could I possibly watch another of my babies go through what Amy had suffered? I waited for Him to explain, but I heard nothing.

By the time Katie was four years old, she was off all the medications. The doctors felt Katie could not have oxalosis. She had not developed one symptom of kidney failure or even the disease. I believe God heard my cries, and He healed her.

Amy loved her baby sister. If she was jealous, we could not tell it. She didn't seem to be bothered by the attention she was getting. I would talk to Amy as I cared for Katie, explaining what I was doing. She would watch for a while, then run off to play.

As I started nursing Katie one day, Amy ran to the bedroom and came back with her doll. She sat down on the floor, pulled her shirt up and started nursing her baby doll. "My baby hungry," she said. I praised her for feeding her baby. She looked so proud sitting there feeding her doll. I knew some day Amy would make a loving and caring mother.

The doctors told us several times there was a good possibility Amy would never be able to have children. They were not even sure what puberty would be like for her. It wasn't something we could even be concerned about. We were still trying to help her live through childhood!

Photos

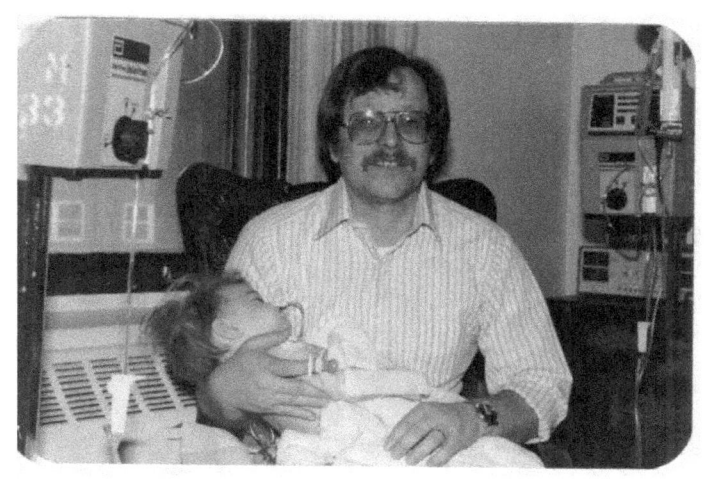

Michael holding Amy after second transplant

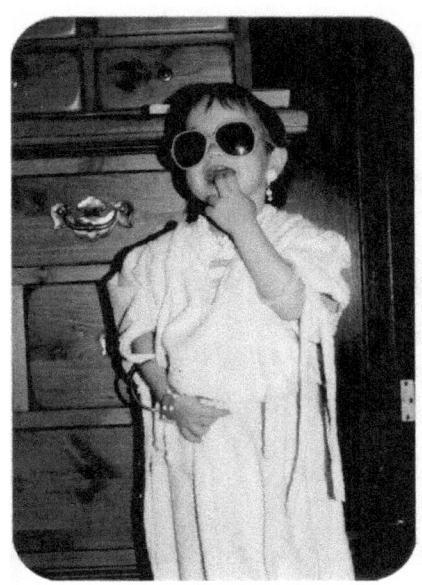

Amy playing dress up

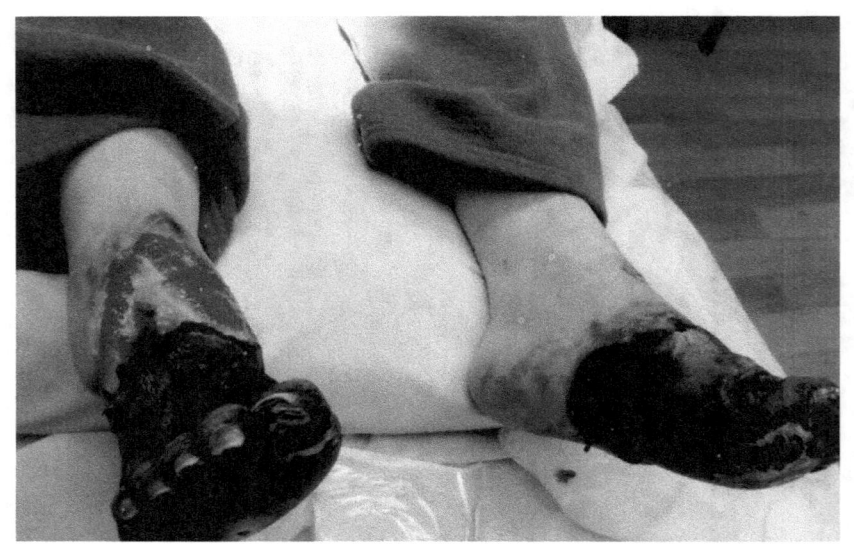

Amy's feet just prior to amputation

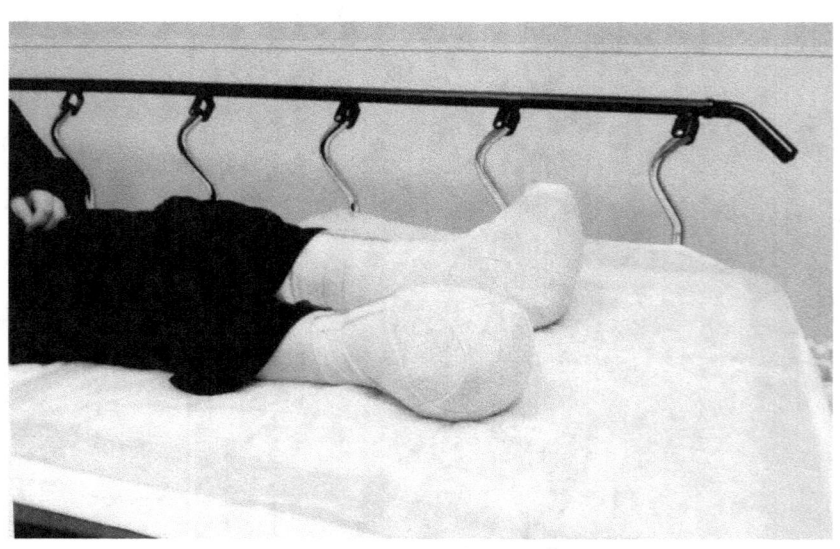

Amy's feet just after amputation

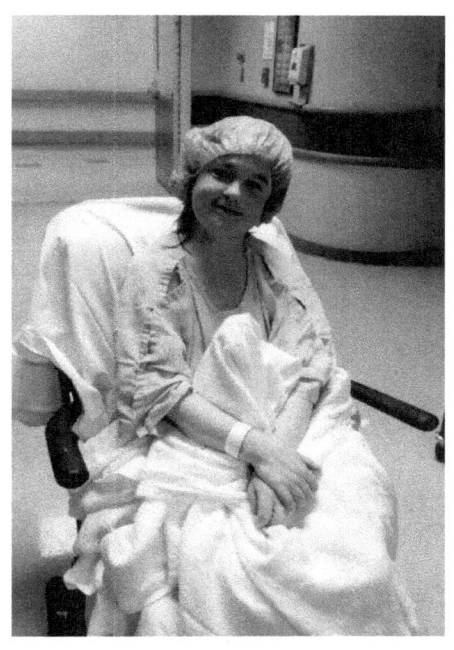

Amy heading to liver transplant surgery

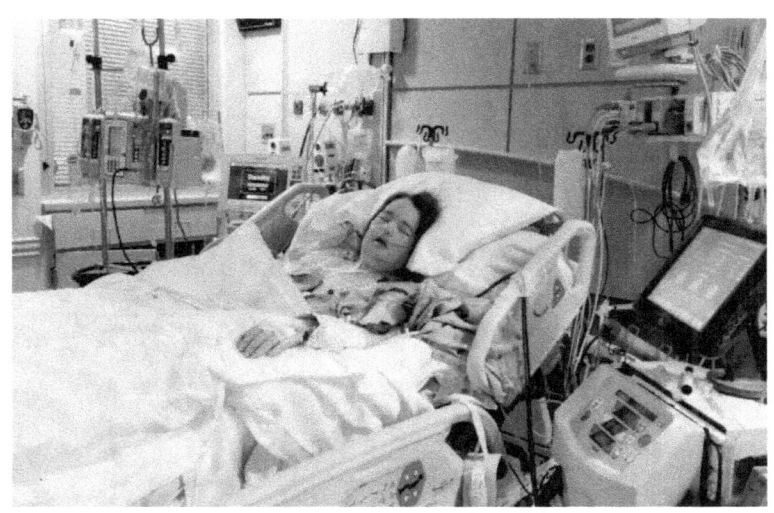

After the liver transplant

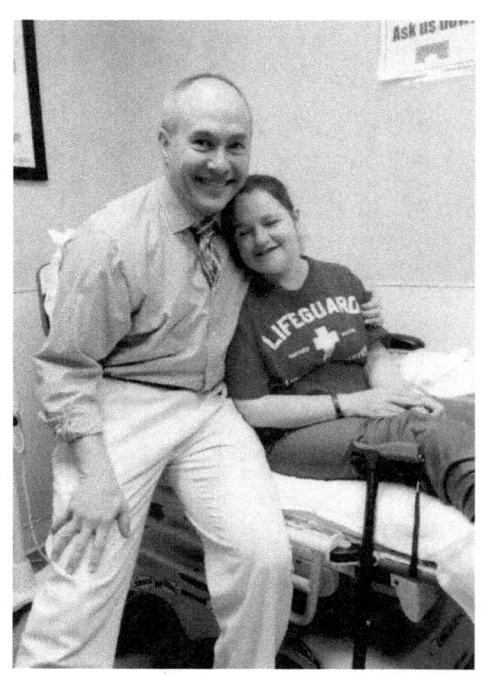

Amy with Dr. Roese

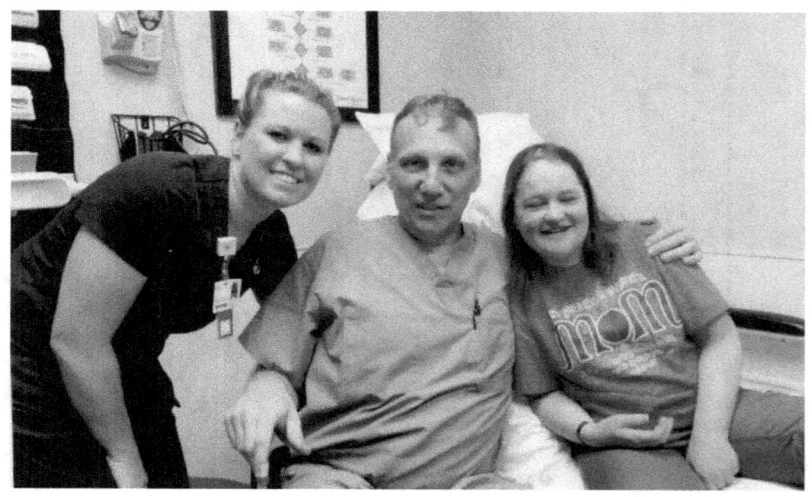

Amy, Dr. Hladik & Nurse Arica

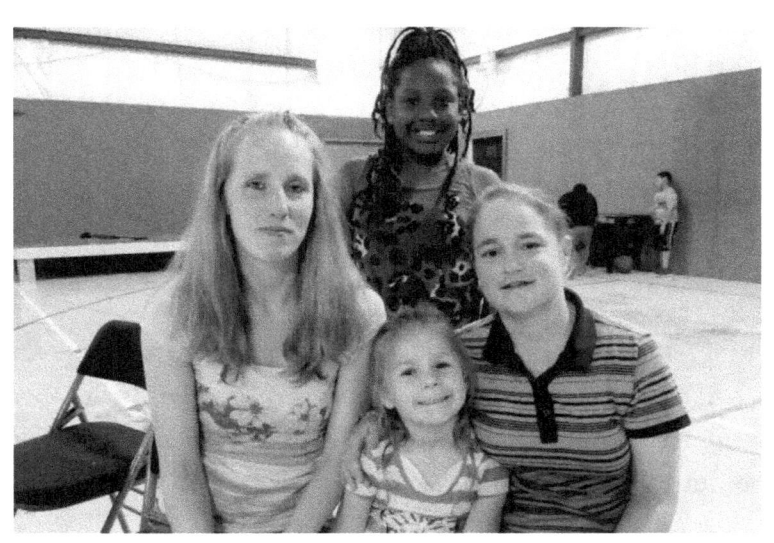

Amy and sisters Katie, Gabriella & Jaelynn

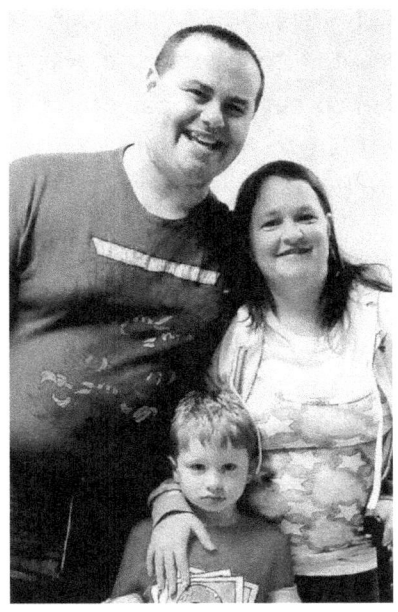

Amy, Matt and Joshua today

Chapter 13

Life at Potter's House

Katie gained weight and grew, as well as Amy, but at a faster rate. Amy continued to have feeding problems. Due to being tube fed, there was not the natural desire to put anything into her mouth. I didn't have to worry that she would put a foreign object into her mouth and choke on it, a very natural activity for small children. Amy simply put nothing in her mouth except liquids.

She had to drink at least 72 ounces of liquid a day to keep her kidney flushed. I was constantly urging her to drink. All the fluid was another factor for her not wanting to eat; she was too full to get hungry. She had to learn to start eating. As she watched me eat, I could tell she was curious. Slowly, I managed to get her to eat some baby food. Chicken and peas were her favorite. I knew she would like other foods if I could just get her to taste them.

One day, I was eating some spaghetti and tried to get her to take a bite. She refused, turning away when the spoon got close to her mouth. Scooping her up in my arms, I pushed a small bite into her mouth, clamped her lips shut and prayed she wouldn't choke before swallowing it. She kicked and squirmed and fought to spit it out. I held on tight to her mouth and prayed harder. Suddenly, a surprise look came upon her face. I let go of her mouth. She had swallowed the spaghetti! I was overjoyed.

"Amy, wasn't that deliciously good?" She smiled and nodded her head. I offered her more; she actually took it and ate it too. As she fed herself the small pieces of spaghetti I cut up, I collapsed in a chair and watched. Forcing the food worked, but it took a lot out of me. I just hoped the next food I introduced wouldn't require such severe tactics.

Except for a flu virus ever so often, Amy was healthy for about 17 months after the transplant. When Katie was five months old, Amy one day began acting out. She was extremely hyper and could not stay focused on anything. I was on the verge of pulling out my hair because she wouldn't listen or obey. It just was not Amy!

I chased her down for the 100th time that day for doing something she knew not to do. Collapsing in a chair, I watched as she darted around the living room, not able to put my finger on the problem. Was it really Amy, or was I setting her off somehow?

She removed her clothing and sped past me. I saw something I had been dreading and trying to avoid. Amy's back had tiny little blisters in several places-chickenpox! It was why she was so hyper and crazy. She just couldn't tell me what was wrong. Her doctor met us at the door of the emergency room and led us to a private room from other patients and their families. She took one look at Amy, confirmed chickenpox and arranged to have her admitted immediately. Chickenpox in transplant patients can potentially be deadly.

Amy was taken to a private room. Of course, I couldn't leave her. Katie was five months old, nursing and couldn't leave me. The nurses took care of the problem. They pulled an extra crib into the room for Katie and the three of us were placed under quarantine! I was not totally confined. If needed, I could come and go because I had chickenpox as a child.

Michael visited us at the hospital throughout our ten-day stay. During the course of the virus, Amy was very ill and even developed encephalitis extending her medical history list. The doctors were on top of it, and Amy came out of the illness no worse off than before the illness. There were many prayers sent up by almost everyone we knew!

Christmas 1986 arrived, and the Potter's House was full. The owners of the house, all the volunteers, Michael and I wanted Christmas to be extra special for the people staying there. Many organizations were involved with the house from the beginning donating materials, money, supplies, anything needed. These organizations also came through at Christmas supplying presents for everyone in the house and their patients in the hospital.

It turned out to be a beautiful Christmas. People from several denominations were staying in the house, including a Jewish family. Elaine and her husband were there with their young son who needed a kidney transplant. They had never celebrated Christmas, but they joined in the celebrations that year. Elaine stayed up all night with me wrapping Christmas presents and helping decide who should get what. I knew this Christmas, like the one in 1984 with Jimmy, would stay in my memory. Many Christmases have come and gone, but none of them could compare to these two.

During the two years we were at the house, Amy made many friends. She enjoyed playing with the children, seemingly understanding when a child was a patient. It was alright with her just to sit with that child if too ill to run around the playroom.

One of her special friends was ten-year-old Johnny who was at the house with his parents waiting on test results. Johnny had a kidney transplant at the age of two and now was in kidney failure again. He also was experiencing signs and symptoms of possible liver failure. Johnny enjoyed talking with Amy, and they would spend a lot of time sitting together. Someone had given him a stuffed bunny, and he allowed Amy to hold it while pretending the bunny talked. She would laugh, hug the bunny and then Johnny. It seemed he thought of her as a little sister.

As the weeks went by, Johnny's condition worsened. He had to be readmitted to the hospital and asked to see Amy before leaving the house. While hugging her, he presented his special bunny. "I have to go to the hospital. Will you take care of my bunny for me?"

She took the bunny and nodded her head. "Yes," she whispered. Johnny then left with his parents for the hospital. That night, Amy insisted on sleeping with the bunny.

Weeks later, Johnny told the hospital chaplain he was ready to die. He was just concerned his mother wasn't ready to let him go. It wasn't the first time seeing a child more concerned about others than their own death, yet it still amazed me! Do these children somehow see and know where they are headed?

Johnny passed away not too long after that conversation with the chaplain. We explained to Amy that

Johnny went to heaven. She responded by getting the bunny out of her bed and rocking it.

I won't know until I can ask Jesus why some survived while others did not. It will be one of the first questions I'll ask Him.

Winter turned into spring, and the girls were both doing great. Amy was walking and talking some. It was obvious she was smart, even with her lack of communication skills. Katie had absolutely no problems from the oxalosis. Her kidney function tests remained normal. She was walking and chasing after her big sister.

I was depressed; I should have been happy. My girls were healthy! Michael was involved in fund raising for the house. He even planned and participated in a bike ride from Minneapolis to North Carolina. He and others, including transplant patients, joined the ride at different spots along the trip. The girls and I took a plane and met him in Indiana for part of the trip. We put the girls in a bike trailer and pulled them a few miles.

I started seeing a therapist who referred me to a psychiatrist. They diagnosed me with several forms of depression-an inherited genetic depression, seasonal, post traumatic, a delayed post-partum and an environmentally induced depression. I was a mess! The doctor prescribed an antidepressant which caused severe drowsiness. I couldn't take care of the girls and consequently stopped taking it after just a couple of weeks.

The therapist recommended we leave the Potter's house. I shouldered the concerns, worries and sorrows of others and needed to get away from all the illness, especially since the girls were doing so well. The long, cold winters in Minnesota were wearing on me too. I needed warmth and sunshine. Michael and I talked it over. We discussed it with the girls' doctor. He felt both girls could be managed in Indiana if we decided to move back.

Amy was four and Katie was 15 months when we packed up and moved back home to Indiana. We purchased a small two-bedroom house in Hope, a small town near Columbus. Once moved, we felt as if we could have a normal life. We were no longer surrounded by families battling major illnesses.

Chapter 14

Life Back in Indiana

It was good being back home, around family and old friends. The girls could visit with Michael's parents, aunts, uncles and cousins. Both girls were happy and healthy. Amy was catching up with other children her age and was excited to start kindergarten in a few months.

Before Amy started school, I took her for a vision exam. We already knew Amy had oxalate crystals in her retinas, but we were not prepared for the exam results. Her retinas were so damaged that she might be legally blind. The optometrist wanted to refer her to the Indiana School for the Blind for a consultation. We agreed even though I felt Amy's vision was better than what he thought.

At the consultation, several people talked with Amy and watched as she played. I also observed the blind students at the school and could not keep from crying as they groped around their surroundings for whatever they needed. They lived in a darkness while never seeing their own reflection, their parents or all the beautiful colors in the world. They lived in the school rather than with their families. The school certainty seemed to be a much needed facility for these little children. They were learning how to survive in a seeing world, but I could never bring myself to send Amy there to live. I was selfish; I wanted her home with me.

After spending time with Amy, the staff met with us to share the results of their testing. They did not believe Amy was legally blind. Her vision was poor, but she could see, well enough to function in most situations.

The following day, the referring eye doctor called and apologized for diagnosing her as legally blind. He had based the diagnosis on the condition of her retinas. He did not know how, but some way Amy was able to see. I knew! God had once more placed His mercy on Amy.

It wasn't her vision I was as concerned with as much as her hearing. Amy just did not pay attention when I was talking. I knew her well enough to know she was very intelligent, but she didn't seem to understand my conversations.

I took Amy for a hearing test. The audiologist afterward explained there was nothing wrong with her hearing. She was just ignoring me! That really angered me. I spent the next week scolding and even spanking her. One day, I spanked her when she seemed to ignore a simple request. She turned to me with a total look of confusion and with words that hurt, "Mommy, I didn't know what you said."

I wrapped my arms around her and cried. Something was not right. I was convinced she wasn't having seizures. It just seemed she couldn't hear. I called and scheduled another hearing appointment, this time at Riley Hospital. This audiologist found a profound hearing loss. Amy needed hearing aids! After taking her history, the audiologist felt Amy had lost her hearing due to meningitis after the first transplant or the use of all the antibiotics. How had the first audiologist missed it? Amy was fitted for hearing aids and adjusted well to them. She was finally able to respond when I spoke to her!

Except for catching the flu and keeping it a little longer than most kids, Amy stayed fairly healthy for several years. When she was 11 years old and in fifth grade, she developed a fever. I took her to the doctor where blood was drawn for cultures. It would take a few days to get the results. The doctor thought she had the flu and sent us home.

At home, her temperature remained up. Amy stayed in my bed and seemed sicker than usual. I knew it was worse than the flu when she had what seemed to be a seizure. Michael and I took her back to the doctor, and Amy collapsed on the office floor. The doctor didn't hesitate in contacting the local hospital to start the admitting process.

Amy's condition worsened over the next two days. Sometimes, she didn't even know she was in the hospital. Her friend, Arica, came to visit Amy with her mother. She woke up and talked coherently for a few minutes with them. She recognized Arica! I hoped this meant improvement, but later the doctor came in with horrible news. Amy was going into kidney failure. She was notifying The University of Minnesota Medical Center. By the time a plan materialized, Amy was in liver and heart failure.

The transplant center decided to send a medical flight to transport Amy to Minnesota. The plane arrived late that day, complete with a doctor and nurses. By that time we had the results of the blood cultures, Amy had pneumococcal virus. Just a few months earlier, the Muppet creator, Jim Henson, died from this virus. He was a healthy individual. Amy was immune suppressed. We were all terrified!

Once the team had her stabilized enough for the flight, Amy was taken by ambulance to the waiting plane. I was allowed to ride on the flight but was squeezed into the tail of the plane, where I couldn't even see Amy. I was given a head set which enabled me to talk to her, and she could hear me.

When we arrived in Minneapolis, we were taken by ambulance from the airport to the hospital. Amy was placed in intensive care. Because her pediatrician had ordered the blood cultures in the beginning, the doctors knew what they were fighting. A couple of days after arriving in Minnesota, I could thankfully see a turn around. Her organs began to improve.

While in the hospital, I asked Amy if she remembered Arica and her mother visiting. She did remember, but wanted to know who the man was in the chair beside her bed while they were there. He had just sat there looking at her and looked really kind. There had not been a man! I had been sitting in it but offered it to Arica and her mom upon their arrival. Neither one sat in it, and no one else did either. In thinking about it, I found that odd. Why had one of us not taken that chair? We all just gathered around the chair. Amy insisted there had been a man sitting there. We concluded it was Jesus.

Amy was discharged from the hospital. All her organs were functioning perfectly, including her kidney. Looking at her, it was amazing how well she looked. We returned home to resume our lives. Amy returned to school. Her teacher, Mr. Webster, presented a song to us he had written. The lyrics are in the back of this book.

I went back to work. There was not a day that went by that I wasn't praying for Amy. Because she had received her first transplant at 15 months, she was unable to have her vaccinations against measles, mumps or rubella. I worried about her being exposed to one of the childhood diseases. I prayed this would not happen, that her kidney would always function perfectly. She stayed well, and her kidney tests always came back normal.

Amy seemed to enjoy school despite the challenges of her hearing and vision loss. Personnel in Flat Rock-Hawcreek School Corporation provided Amy with whatever she needed to succeed. She was given special equipment in order to hear the teacher's voice. Amy would wear earphones and the teacher a microphone. At the end of class, she would collect the equipment and take it to the next class. The vision consultant ordered large print books for Amy. They were really big books, and I thought some of them might have weighed more than her!

I worried that Amy would rebel at all the things that made her different from her classmates, especially as she entered middle and high school. Like everything else in her life, Amy took all the necessary differences in stride. She was a very determined child and worked extremely hard to accomplish whatever was asked of her.

Throughout her years in high school, Amy continued to be appreciated by the teachers for her work ethic. Her friends and classmates were accepting and provided a great support system. She never complained about being bullied. I believe Amy was touched by God and received a personality that enabled her to deal with things that would cause others to collapse.

When Amy was 18 and a senior in high school, severe illness hit again. She started having high temperatures and was admitted to the hospital. The testing didn't reveal anything. Once more, we were off to Minnesota. Michael drove us. Katie remained with friends.

Amy lay in the back seat and slept. Whenever we made a bathroom stop, I would help her out of the car and to the rest room. She would vomit every time. Michael and I were so concerned.

It took 18 long hours before we arrived at the hospital! By the time Amy was admitted, she had an odd blister type of rash on the back of her leg. The doctors decided to biopsy and culture the area. When the results came back, we learned she had a herpes simplex virus, the virus that caused mouth sores. Because she was immune suppressed due to the kidney transplant, the virus had spread throughout her body. Soon, Amy was covered with blisters from head to toe and was miserable. The doctors began treatment.

Michael was able to stay with us. He and I stayed at the local Ronald McDonald House. Sadly, the organ transplant house we had managed was closed.

When Amy's virus cleared up enough that we could manage it with oral meds, we drove back home. We had been home just a few days when Amy complained that her leg was hurting. When looking at it, I discovered it was swollen, cold and blue-typical signs of a blood clot. I called her doctor who told me to take her to the emergency room. Amy was as big as me, but I managed to carry her out of the house and to the car.

At the emergency room, an ultrasound of the leg proved she did have a blood clot which extended from her ankle to her pelvis. Treatment was started to dissolve it. Everyone was concerned about the clot reaching the kidney. An internal medicine doctor was consulted, and he took over Amy's care.

Amy was sick of being in the hospital. She was miserable and depressed. The doctor sent her home after just a couple of days. She needed Heparin shots which were administered directly into the abdominal muscle by me, her own in-home nurse. The injections were painful. She cried every time receiving one; I cried with her. She was miserable. Amy just wanted her life back! She was anxious to return to school.

Graduation was in a few months! Afterward, she planned to enroll at Ivy Tech Community College. The blood clot was interfering with plans for her life.

The Heparin injections did their work and dissolved the blood clot. When the shots were discontinued, we both rejoiced. Amy was so tired of getting the painful injections, and it broke my heart to stick her. She returned to school, but her leg continued to swell and be painful at times. According to the doctor, she should expect that reaction for the rest of her life. She took that information in stride; she would just deal with it!

When Amy graduated in June of 2002 from Hauser High School, she enrolled that fall for part-time classes at Ivy Tech. She attended classes for Early Childhood Education and started a job at a day care. After working at that job for about a year, she opened her own day care, Amy's Kids, in the basement of our home. She treated the children as if they were her own. Amy loved them, and they loved her in return. She had found her niche in life!

Chapter 15

A Nightmare Revealed

For the next three years, Amy did not have any health problems. But, she began to complain about having difficulty concentrating. Her school work and grades began to suffer. She was moody, and Katie reported that Amy was acting like a five-year-old at times.

One evening after I had gone to bed, Amy came to me crying. She was upset but couldn't tell me why. I scooted over, and she climbed in bed with me. It was if she was a very young child. She was shaking, didn't seem able to talk. Suddenly, she arched her neck, threw her head back and went into what I thought was a grand mal seizure. I screamed for Michael. By the time he came, the seizure was over even though Amy was still not acting right. Her eyes kept rolling back in her head, and she was mumbling incoherently. We had no choice but to head to the hospital.

She was examined and tests were performed. Nothing could be found that explained the seizure. In fact, there was not even a seizure according to the tests. I knew better; I knew what a grand mal seizure looked like! The doctor just looked at me as if I were just another distraught mother and discharged her.

Throughout the night, Amy continued to have the seizures while in my bed. She would arch her back so far that I was concerned she would break her neck. Her speech was garbled; her eyes would roll back. After hours of this behavior,

I was afraid she was going to die. We returned to the emergency room.

The doctor admitted her. Throughout the next couple of days, Amy continued to have the seizures as well as the other behaviors. The doctors were puzzled! They started talking about psychological problems. Amy persisted in acting very childlike and didn't want me to leave. The staff informed me, through their observations, that she seemed to only have the seizure-like activity when I was around. If I left, then she would not have another one until I returned. This really concerned me. Was I the cause of Amy's problems?

A psychiatrist was consulted. She talked with Amy alone. After the interview, the psychiatrist talked with me and praised Amy. She felt we had a very good relationship and didn't feel Amy had any psychological problems. This made me feel better, but we were no closer to determining the problem. Amy didn't exactly know how to explain these episodes, only that she was experiencing strange feelings and seeing things that were not there.

Amy was transferred to Indiana University Hospital. She was placed on the seizure unit and observed 24 hours a day. Amy displayed the same behaviors, and the neurologists asked if she had ever been molested. The patterns they were seeing were found in girls and young women who had been molested. Amy had never been sexually molested. I knew! As close as I was to her, I would have known. Besides, Amy would have shared with me! I had always been very careful where my girls went and who they were around. I didn't even discuss this with Amy; I felt the doctors were looking in the wrong direction.

They discharged her. We went home, still not knowing what was causing this strange behavior. Everything had been done-EEG's, cat scans of the brain and anything else the doctors could think of to do. We would see a local neurologist if the pseudo seizures persisted, false seizures caused by an emotional problem.

Michael and I didn't know what to think. Had all her health problems and the way we handled them caused emotional problems? Amy had always appeared so resilient. She always bounced back from everything.

She continued the bizarre behaviors. Gradually, Amy began to talk after the episodes. At first, she kept seeing a particular male medical professional that we had taken her to from the age of four until six. I will refer to the man as Dr. Brown.

Amy began to cry during her trances. I would ask her what was happening, where she was and who was there. Over the next few weeks, she revealed that during her appointment Dr. Brown would molest her, what he did to her and what she was wearing. I would remember the clothing. Amy normally did not remember the clothing she had as a young child, and we did not have pictures of her in those outfits. There had to be truth in her story.

This man would request I stay in the waiting room with Katie. All the parents waited there. The assistant would reassure me that she would be fine. All her life, I turned her over to medical personnel. Amy and I had been conditioned, and this man took advantage. Pedophiles always know who they can choose as their victims.

After one visit, Amy had fought him and bit him. Then he bit her back really hard. When asking why I had not noticed the bite, she reminded me that I had and questioned her. He always threatened Amy not to tell.

My memory of this bite mark returned. She claimed Katie was responsible. Katie was two at the time. I was shocked that Katie would bite her sister and spanked her. Katie denied it and cried. I never once considered that she had gotten the bite earlier at Dr. Brown's office! Tears flowed down my face. I had wrongly spanked my baby; my other daughter had been violated!

Amy had always loved to wear dresses until suddenly not wanting to wear them. When getting her ready to go to Dr. Brown's office, she would want to wear long pants and long sleeves even in the summer. Sadly, I made her wear the dress; I had made it easy for him to molest her. Dr. Brown would instruct her to throw the panties away as soon as she got home. I recalled that her panties use to disappear. Since they were so small, I always thought they went down the washer drain with all the tiny socks.

Amy disclosed how Dr. Brown use to nibble on her chin and neck. Now I understood Amy's reaction when I tried to nibble on her chin. Katie and I were in bed one day playing. I was nibbling on her chin and ears, and she was laughing. Amy came in and climbed in bed with us. I grabbed her and started nibbling on her chin, trying to tickle her. She became hysterical and started screaming; she jumped off the bed still screaming at me. I didn't understand her negative reaction then.

Amy always hated the nursery song "Hush Little Baby-Mama's Gonna Buy You A Mocking Bird." I could never understand until she finally revealed why. Dr. Brown would hum this song as he molested her. If Amy happened to hear that song, she would go into a trance and her eyes would roll back into her head. I was furious with this man. I asked God why He allowed it. Why didn't He stop it? How could I have not known? How could my little girl be violated without me recognizing it? I always assured myself that if my girls were ever molested, I would know. But, I missed it! I hated Dr. Brown, but I also hated myself for placing Amy in that situation.

Amy reassured me that it wasn't my fault, that I couldn't have known. She could not share with me; Dr. Brown would not allow it. He would tell Amy that I brought her there for him to do that because of being bad. I now understood why Amy would ask if she was being good during her early school years. Amy knew if she wasn't being good that I would take her to him. Even if she was good, I would still take her-just not as frequently.

My heart ached knowing what she had been through. Had I walked in on him molesting Amy, there is no doubt in my mind I would have killed him. His assistants would not have been able to stop me. I would have attacked him and bitten his face off; I would have clawed his eyes out. Even now, after all these year, I want to attack him. What would have happened had I killed him? It was actually good I didn't know. I would have gone to prison, unable to raise my girls.

I began to research a therapist for Amy. I found a really good one. She had lots of experience in working with pseudo seizures with regression resulting from sexual molestation.

She believed Amy had been molested by Dr. Brown explaining that young girls try to forget the incidents. They tend to box it off somewhere in their minds, forgetting it temporarily. Eventually, something triggers the memories, and they can start regressing and reliving the incidents. This is what happened to Amy.

She also diagnosed Amy with Dissociative Identity Disorder (DID) or split personality. Amy had two personalities, herself and a young child about five years old. For some time, we had noticed Amy had periods of acting very immature. The episodes were brief, easy to overlook. When checking her school assignments, I could now understand why some were so bad that she had to redo them. Her instructor pointed out some of her assignment looked as if a young child had done them. Once more, I was angry at myself. Why didn't I notice this all along?

Her therapist asked me to take Amy to a psychiatrist. The psychiatrist supported the diagnosis of DID resulting from sexual molestation. She confirmed that Amy had two personalities, but that DID usually resulted in three personalities. She asked if I had ever seen the third personality.

On the drive home as Amy napped, I thought over the comments of the psychiatrist. Cases like Amy's were complex. It would take years and years of therapy for Amy to get over this, if ever. I prayed during the drive, asking God for His help and how to help her deal with two personalities.

Suddenly, I realized Amy did have a third personality. I hadn't seen it but a few times, always shocked. Amy would become furious and would attack verbally with curse words that I didn't even know she knew. Her voice was gruff. It startled and even frightened me. Afterward, Amy acted like it didn't even happen. Normally, she never used curse words; so, I just let the episodes slide and forgot about them.

Dr. Brown not only molested Amy, but messed with her mind. He created problems that might never be fixable; he created problems for our entire family. We chose to start the process of criminally charging him. I knew Amy could not be his only victim. She mentioned that sometimes he molested another child while she was in the room.

I began my own investigation and called Dr. Brown's office to obtain Amy's file. A new assistant gave me the name of another assistant who worked there when Amy was a patient. I remembered her. She had carried Amy out to me a couple of times. Amy had been crying, covered with perspiration and refusing to walk. When asking her why Amy was so upset, she suggested Amy was just upset from the procedures. Amy wouldn't talk about it. The second time she came out that distraught, I transferred Amy's care to another office. I didn't realize what I was rescuing Amy from. Three years with Dr. Brown, however, had done its damage!

I traced the assistant down and called her on the phone and asked specific questions, in particular if assistants remained with the patient during care. Usually they did, but sometimes they would leave, such as when developing x-rays. I also asked if she ever felt anything odd took place in the office.

She responded in a way that made me wonder if she really did suspect something.

Amy and I went to see a police detective. I explained what we had learned. He said it was challenging to develop a case 15 years after the crime, but he would check into it. When we didn't hear from him after a couple of weeks, I called. He couldn't find any evidence to support our claim. No complaints had ever been lodged against Dr. Brown. The detective had interviewed the assistant, and she stated the assistants never left the patient. However, people would often change their story thinking they might be accused. We would need evidence or other people claiming the same charges in order to prosecute.

I decided to find evidence. Somewhere, there were other people he molested, and I was determined to find them. Over the next two years, I talked to people who had heard rumors. People knew other people that had suddenly stopped taking their kids to him. I was able to track down one such mother, but she refused to meet to discuss it.

I couldn't understand how this man could get away with this. He was well-known and one of the top doctors in his field. Was he being protected by someone? Why hadn't somebody complained about him? Or, was it possible they had with nothing being done as in Amy's case? Why wouldn't mothers speak to me about it? I think they were afraid to find out he molested their child. It was easier to ignore!

During those two years while I was talking with people treated by Dr. Brown, Amy was talking with God. She was determined to get over it and started going to a Bible study for young adults. She faithfully read her Bible and listened to sermons by Joyce Meyer. One day, Amy stressed that God wanted us to forgive. She was going to forgive Dr. Brown and just go on with her life.

Over the following two years as I watched Amy, it was obvious God had healed her. We were no longer seeing the other personalities. The pseudo seizures stopped. She could even listen to the mocking bird song without freaking out. What usually took therapy many years to cure, God and forgiveness healed in just a few.

If Amy could forgive Dr. Brown, then I needed to forgive too. By forgiving, our entire family could let go of the hurt and move on into the lives God wanted for us.

Chapter 16

Amy's Adult Life

As the years went by, I became very proud of the young woman Amy became-a very loving, caring person who put God first. Medically, she conquered something that had taken the lives of many. Emotionally, she had come through problems causing others to commit suicide. Amy, somehow remained happy and optimistic.

Throughout their lives, I prayed for my daughters' future husbands. I wanted good men for them, men who loved Christ and who would love the girls for who they were. I was especially concerned for Amy. She needed a husband that would accept her vision and hearing deficits and who could deal with her medical issues, a man who could care for her when ill and who would have the faith when faith was demanded. He would need a good Christian family as support during times of stress. If he could love her even half as much as I loved her, then she would be well taken care of. Where do you find such a young man? I knew God would find a way.

By the time Amy had gotten her life back together and no longer needed a therapist, she still had not met the right man. Her dad suggested she join an online dating service. She joined and began meeting young men, but none of them worked out. After almost a year, she was ready to give up. The dating service offered her an opportunity to see matches they had found. She tried one more time and found a young man who lived in Ohio, about two hours away from us.

Matt's credentials sounded too good. He was the same age, worked at a home improvement store and had a college degree in computers. His father was a minister, and Matt wanted to be a minister. Amy was upfront about all her medical problems. He came to our house to meet her and us. Their first date was spent walking around a festival at our small town, Heritage Days. Amy liked him.

The next visit, Amy rode with him to church. They were to go out for lunch afterwards. I decided to call Amy's cell phone to check on them. After all, I reasoned, we didn't really know anything about this man. Amy didn't answer her phone after several attempts. I began to panic. My imagination took over thinking this stranger had kidnapped our daughter, doing no telling what to her! I became more agitated and kept calling. Finally, she answered. I demanded to know where they were. She was just leaving church. I had forgotten that she was taking a class at church after the service. Matt had attended it with her! She laughed when I mentioned kidnapping concerns and told me not to worry. Matt was very nice, and they were going out for the afternoon. I felt like a fool!

When they returned, he stayed and visited with us. We all had a good laugh about the kidnapping. He asked for permission to see her again the next weekend. He even had manners. I liked this young man!

Over the next year and a half, they saw each other every weekend. Matt would come to our house and sleep on our sofa; the next weekend Amy would go to Ohio and stay at his parents' house. Amy repeated to Matt everything concerning her health and even what Dr. Brown did and how it affected her. I was afraid this would be enough to chase him off; he kept coming back. I guess you can't chase off somebody sent by God!

As they began to talk about marriage, I talked with Matt about what marrying Amy entailed. I wanted him to know exactly what to expect; I didn't want him to have any surprises. If he could accept the medical issues, then I could be assured he would take good care of her. He understood. The wedding date was set!

Amy began to make plans to move to Ohio. She and Matt rented an apartment, and she began to move her things there. I struggled with Amy being in another state, where I would not be able to make medical observations. Sometimes, I knew she was ill even before she did! Amy stressed that we didn't have to worry, that we had helped her grow into a strong, independent woman.

On July 11, 2009, Amy and Matt were married. Matt's father, David Steward, performed the ceremony and did an excellent job. It was a beautiful wedding! God answered my prayers concerning my daughter's husband. Matt was a good man who obviously loved Amy. He would see that she got good medical care. Most importantly, he would trust God to take care of her and would turn to Him to intervene during any medical crisis.

In December 2011, Amy became pregnant. This was something her doctors didn't really believe would happen and even hoped it wouldn't happen due to her medical issues. They suggested termination. Amy refused! She had prayed for this baby and was trusting God.

The pregnancy was not without complications. Amy prayed through each problem, and they would be resolved. On August 11, 2012, Joshua Aaron Steward was born four weeks early due to preeclampsia. He weighed 4 pounds 12 ounces. Despite his premature arrival, he did not have any problems and remained in the hospital only one extra day. Joshua was our second grandson. Katie married in 2006. She and her husband, Chris, blessed us with Jayden in 2007.

When the pediatrician started to circumcise Joshua, he could not perform the procedure because Joshua had an abnormality called Megaurethra. This condition could result in many complications such as infection, infertility and cancer among others. Amy and Matt refused to accept this diagnosis. Michael and I took the matter to our church the following Sunday. Our pastor along with church members prayed that Joshua would be normal. When Amy took the baby to a urologist a few weeks later, the doctor told Amy he didn't know what the pediatrician was talking about because Joshua was normal. Joshua was finally circumcised when he was six months old. God was still answering prayers!

I loved watching Amy holding her son. God had been so wonderful to us. Amy was alive, healthy and had a normal life. Now, she had the one thing many doctors thought impossible, a perfect baby from a body that had been through so much.

Chapter 17

A New Nightmare

Shortly after Joshua was born, I kept having a dream that Amy was ill. She was in the hospital, and I was telling Michael we had to go through "this" again. I would wake up upset and wonder why I kept dreaming this dreadful idea. Amy was healthy; her labs were good; she surely wasn't going to need to go through another transplant!

Three months after Joshua was born, Matt called to say Amy was ill. He was taking her to the hospital. Michael and I quickly left for Ohio. Matt met us at the hospital entrance and gave us Amy's room number. He took Michael to get a cup of coffee from the canteen, but I wanted to see Amy and rushed to the room.

As I entered the room, Amy was talking with a doctor. The doctor was telling Amy the results from her blood tests. Her creatinine was 2.4. It had always been normal, 1.0 or below. The doctor didn't know what was causing the rise, but some other tests also indicated probable kidney failure.

Hearing these words, my head began to spin. I started to feel nauseous and backed out of the room searching for a restroom. Michael and Matt were in the hall, and I repeated what the doctor stated. They hurried to her room, and I hurried to the restroom. Bending over the toilet, my mind went back to 1983 when the doctor told us Amy was in kidney failure. My head kept swimming, and I vomited. This couldn't be happening again. Amy had just given birth; she needed to be healthy to raise her little boy!

Amy was discharged and instructed to follow up with her nephrologist. Until the reason for the elevated creatinine was learned, nothing could be done about the test results.

Over the next few months, her creatinine continued to slowly rise. The doctors thought that the problem was probably due to a reoccurrence of the oxalate in the kidney. We refused to believe it. Why would the kidney work for 27 years and then suddenly have crystals accumulate again? Amy's nephrologist also doubted it but couldn't find any other reason for the elevation in her lab results. He sent her to Ohio State University for a kidney biopsy.

When the biopsy results came back, they were inconclusive-no rejection and not enough crystals that would lead to kidney failure. The Minnesota Transplant Center was consulted, and it was determined Amy should return there for an examination.

Amy, Matt and Joshua left for Minnesota at the end of June 2013. I was unable to accompany them. We had adopted two little girls who were 2 and 8, and I felt I needed to stay and care for them. Matt's parents went to help care for Joshua while Amy was undergoing tests.

Another kidney biopsy was performed. There were minimal crystals in the kidney, but the kidney did have some chronic rejection. The doctors decided to change her immunosuppressant drugs. Two days after starting the medication, Amy complained her legs were hurting. She was assured it was expected and the symptoms would improve.

They returned home on new meds, but still without a definitive answer to the slowly worsening kidney failure. The doctors believed she probably had another two years before needing another transplant.

Amy continued on with life, taking care of Joshua and dealing with the leg pain caused by the new drugs. Each time she reported this to the doctors, they would reassure her the symptoms were to be expected.

On August 12th, Matt called. Amy legs were hurting and turning blue. Her family physician had taken one look at her leg discoloration and told her to go straight to the emergency room. Matt called back later. She had been admitted to ICU, and her creatinine was 9.0, an alarming jump from the 2.7 when she had been in Minnesota.

Katie came to care for the girls, and Michael and I left for Ohio. Arriving at the hospital, we discovered Amy was being transferred to another hospital where she could receive more intensive care. Once she was moved there, she was taken to surgery. A catheter was placed in her chest which went to her heart so she could receive dialysis treatments through it. Then, she was started on emergency dialysis.

Over the following week, her condition improved. Her legs became pink again and quit hurting. The doctors said she would have to remain on dialysis.

Matt had just started a new job. He could not figure out how he would get her to dialysis. Amy couldn't drive even if she felt like taking herself to the dialysis clinic. He could not take off from a job just started. Amy and Joshua would stay in Indiana so I could transport her to dialysis.

It was a sad situation. Amy wanted to be with her husband, and he wanted her there. But, there were no better options. Matt would come every weekend to see her and Joshua. Until we could figure out what we needed to do about Amy's health, this was how we had to live. We just believed it would be temporary, that things would turn around.

I moved two-year-old Jaelynn's toddler bed into our room. A crib and a twin bed was put in her room for Amy and Joshua. I left the baby monitor in the room so I could hear if Amy needed me or wasn't able to get up and care for Joshua.

Amy returned to her former internist for care. The social worker from the hospital in Ohio set up dialysis treatments at a center in Greensburg, 20 minutes from us. Her labs indicated she only needed dialysis two days a week. I drove her there on Mondays and Fridays.

In late September, Amy began having worse problems with her legs. Lab tests showed her potassium was elevated, and the doctor thought that was causing the leg pain. He put her on dialysis three times a week. She went Monday, Wednesday and Friday but continued to believe the new medications were causing the leg problems and the elevated potassium.

We weren't sure what to do. None of us believed it was the oxalosis. She had been to several doctors, but no one could pinpoint what was causing the kidney failure. Each doctor had their own opinion but unable to prove their possible diagnosis; so, each one came back to the oxalosis theory.

On Sunday, November 3rd, Amy was up most of the night with severe leg pain. About 4 a.m., I drove her to the hospital emergency room. Her legs and feet were so painful she could hardly walk. The ER doctor had lab work done and found her potassium to be very elevated. He ordered a dialysis treatment at the center and gave no explanation for the severe leg pain.

I took her to the dialysis center. The nurse hooked her up and started dialysis. I left to run some errands while she dialyzed. Less than an hour later, Amy called me to come pick her up. She was in so much pain she couldn't sit still and had asked the nurse to take her off. I took her home. Amy crawled to the bed because her legs were hurting so much. I called her primary physician but couldn't get an appointment until the next day.

The next morning, she was examined and found to be very dehydrated. The doctor sent her to the hospital to receive IV fluids. After getting the fluids, her legs were still hurting terribly. So, I borrowed a wheelchair and wheeled her back to the emergency room. The doctor found the potassium level to be even higher and ordered dialysis. We were both reprimanded because she hadn't finished her dialysis treatment the day before. Amy had been hurting so much she couldn't even sit still for the treatment! I asked the doctor what she would have done in the same situation. She didn't have an answer but prescribed medication to help bring Amy's potassium down. I hoped that would help with the pain!

We returned home. Amy cried in pain the rest of the evening. She climbed in bed with me that night, and we both stayed awake. I pleaded with God to take the pain away. I quoted every scripture I could think of about healing, but the pain continued. At 4 a.m., I got up emotionally exhausted from all the trips to the doctor, ER and dialysis and from watching Amy suffer. I woke Michael and asked him to take her back to ER and somehow make them understand that something had to be done. Michael carried her, and I helped get her into the car.

Two hours later, Michael called to say she was being admitted. Finally, they had given her pain medicine. After three trips to the ER, something was being done!

Katie came over to stay with Jaelynn. After I had taken Gabby to school, I went to the hospital. Amy was being given IV pain medicine which helped to some degree. She was also going to dialysis. I called Matt and let him know she had been admitted, and he immediately left Ohio to be with her.

Over the next two days, Amy still remained in pain in spite of receiving strong narcotics. Amy's lab tests revealed an elevated troponin level which indicated a possible heart attack. In addition, the tests showed she had a bundle blockage in her heart. The reason her legs hurt were because the blood vessels were having spasms preventing the blood from circulating. The doctor felt this was also occurring in her heart causing a heart attack. He thought the problem was related to oxalate crystals that had accumulated in her blood vessels, and he would need to consult with a cardiologist.

The cardiologist then ordered more heart tests. I don't think Amy was even aware of what was happening due to all the narcotics she was receiving. When the results were obtained, the cardiologist determined she had not had a heart attack, that the troponin level was elevated due to the other factors.

On Friday, a doctor came in to look at her feet because they had started turning blue. He called in a vascular surgeon, Dr. Jason Christy. Amy would need to go to surgery to have dye placed in her veins through a catheter placed in her groin. This dye would enable him to look at her veins and see what was interrupting the blood flow to her feet. Amy was now aware and very upset because the kidney doctor indicated contrast dye would harm the kidney. She was still hoping the kidney would recover as soon as it was determined what was causing it to fail.

Dr. Christy explained that the kidney wasn't working because the oxalate crystals were accumulating in her blood vessels creating a blockage. It could possibly be something else, but we needed to know the cause so the problem could be fixed. He would use carbon dioxide first. If that didn't make the blood vessels visible, he would have to switch to the dye. Amy, Matt, Michael and I discussed it and agreed with the plan. Dr. Christy would schedule the procedure, hoping it could wait until Monday.

In the meantime, all we could do was pray the blood circulation to her feet would resume quickly. The next day, Dr. Christy examined her feet; her legs were now starting to turn blue. She needed to go to surgery for the procedure without delay. If something wasn't done quickly, Amy could lose both her legs. Matt signed the surgery consent form, and Dr. Christy left to make arrangements. Michael called our pastors, Mark and Dona Owings, who came to the hospital to pray with Amy.

Amy was taken to surgery, and we were left to wait and pray. After the procedure, we were called to a room to consult with the surgeon. Dr. Christy along with his partner, Dr.

Douglas Roese, met with us to discuss their findings. We could tell by their faces that things were not good. Amy's blood vessels were blocked from the waist down, and they thought that spasms were causing the vessels to close. They had tried carbon dioxide but ended up having to use the dye to get a better view of the blood vessels. The catheter was left in her groin because it would be necessary to take her back to surgery the next day to see if the vessels had opened up any farther. Amy was going to ICU to have splints placed on her legs to prevent catheter movement. She would be strapped down so she would not be able to pull the catheter out. Dr. Roese felt the situation was very critical. Amy would probably lose her legs. She could very well die. More would be known after the procedure was repeated the next day. The only thing he knew to do was pray. We assured him we were doing just that.

Once we told Pastor Mark what the doctors said, he left and called church members to meet him at church. They gathered there to lift Amy up in prayer.

Amy was admitted to ICU, strapped down and sedated. I knew if she was aware she couldn't move she would panic. A dialysis machine was brought into her room, and dialysis was performed there. Michael went home to be with the kids, and Matt and I sat at her bedside. Matt paced the small room while I held her hand. We both prayed nonstop. We did not want Amy to die. If she did, she would be in heaven, but we knew Amy very much wanted to raise her son. That's what we wanted too. Her legs were both blue and cold while her left foot looked and felt like a block of ice. It would take a miracle to restore the circulation!

The next day, Amy went back to surgery to repeat the procedure. Dye was injected through the catheter into her blood vessels so the doctors could see if there was any improvement. When we met with them afterwards, they said her vessels were somewhat better. The vessels were only blocked above her knees. Things were still critical, but Dr. Roese was a little more optimistic. He wanted to repeat the procedure the next day hoping for even more improvement but cautioned that she could still lose her legs, even her life

Amy returned to ICU, still strapped down and sedated. She wasn't aware we were there, interceding for her in prayer.

The following day, Sunday, the procedure was repeated a third time. The doctors came out this time with smiles on their faces. The blockage had receded even farther; however, her left leg vessels were still blocked. Dr. Roese said she would lose part of her left leg, how much of it he didn't know yet. The next couple of days would tell.

Back to ICU she went. Matt and I remained at her bedside. Amy always enjoyed listening to a healing CD by Gloria Copland. Matt put it on so she could hear it even though we were not sure if she was aware of anything going on around her.

Every so often, Matt or I would raise the sheet and look at her foot. It remained cold and white, apparently due to no circulation to it. I stood by her bed, my hand on her shoulder, listening to the CD. Gloria explained that healing was in our hands and to lay our hands on the sick and take the healing for that person. I wanted my daughter well and said, "I take the blood circulation back for Amy."

After a few minutes, I raised the sheet. Pink lines were running down her leg and into her foot. I touched her foot, and it was warmer. Matt came over to the bed and looked. Suddenly, we were both giddy with excitement. We began praising God and thanking Jesus. We must have caused a disturbance because the nurse came in. She looked at Amy's foot and ran back out of the room.

She returned with Dr. Roese. He looked at her foot, felt it, then looked at us and asked, "What did you do? Did you give her something?"

I don't know what he thought we might have given her or why he even asked that, but we assured him we hadn't given her anything.

He said, "This is amazing!" He left the room and returned with his surgical nurse.

"Look at this, amazing," was all he seemed to be able to say.

The next day, Amy was moved to a regular room. She became more alert and started talking to us. She couldn't remember anything from the previous three days.

Chapter 18

The Nightmare Continues

Over the next four days, Amy continued to improve. Her feet stayed warm and were turning pink. The doctors were all convinced the vascular spasms were caused by the oxalate accumulation in the blood vessels. The kidney doctor consulted with the Minnesota Transplant Center. After much discussion, it was decided that Amy should have dialysis six days a week, five hours a day. This was to clear the crystals from her blood. Most kidney failure patients have dialysis three days a week for three hours at a time. Amy was devastated. That was a lot of dialysis. She felt that it wasn't the oxalate but the new medications that had caused the spasms. The doctor stopped the new medications, only because he felt they weren't needed because the kidney wasn't working any way.

On Sunday, November 17, Amy's feet began to turn blue and became very painful again. We watched in horror as the previous situation seemed to be repeating. Dr. Roese came in and examined her feet and announced the spasms were reoccurring.

"This can't be happening," I told God. "You healed her; she has to stay well!"

But over the next three days, things became worse. The nurses shared that Dr. Roese stayed on the computer and the phone for hours trying to find a solution to stop the spasms. There didn't seem to be an answer anywhere. The hospital staff called a meeting with our family, the doctors, nurses, social workers and everybody involved in her care. The meeting was scheduled in her room so she could be involved, but Amy was on so much pain medication that she wasn't aware anyone was there, let alone what we were discussing.

Dr. Roese led the discussion, what he thought was happening and that he didn't know what else to do. At the least, Amy would lose her feet, possibly her legs. At the worst, she could die.

As a family, we let them know we wanted done whatever could be done. Amy wanted to live. She had a 15-month old baby to raise. When the meeting ended, we didn't know anything more than we had known. Everybody in the room just looked sad.

Later that evening, Dr. Roese returned and talked with Matt and me. He was going to prescribe Viagra. It was a drug for male impotence, even though it originally was developed for use in premature infants for circulation problems. He hoped that by Amy taking it that her circulation would improve. Within two days of starting the drug, her feet became warmer and began turning pink.

On November 22, I was sitting with Amy and praying. I was exhausted. Amy's feet had improved but suddenly things got worse. Her feet hurt; they were still not normal; her toes were purple. Why was she having to go through this again? The only answer was something I had heard years earlier. When a person gets healed, satan will try to return and cause worse problems than before. I didn't know, but maybe that was the reason.

Matt left to get something to eat. Amy began talking. She started telling me things she wanted me to do for Joshua, how to care for him. Then, she kept saying strange, nonsense things like not to let him date wild girls when older.

"Amy, why are you saying this?" I asked.

"Because I want you to take care of him!"

"You have to take care of him, Amy. He needs his mother."

I was afraid Amy was giving up, letting me know she was going to die. She rambled on about Joshua. I felt my heart breaking and began to cry. Amy had suffered so much the past few weeks. I didn't want her to die, but, more than that, I didn't want her to suffer. It hurt more to watch her suffer in pain than to let her go. I wanted her to raise Joshua, but it sure sounded as if she was giving up. As I sat there crying, several of our church members arrived. They gathered around Amy and prayed. One of the women put her arms around me and held me. It is hard to describe what that moment meant. They stayed until Matt arrived.

I was so tired and sad and needed to leave. Amy had been very confused, and maybe Matt could talk with her. I kissed Amy, told her I loved her and then left. All the way home, I cried while praying and asking God to intervene and do something to help Amy.

When arriving home, Michael wanted to know what was happening. I explained how Amy was talking, that I was afraid she was giving up. For the second time in our married life, I saw my husband in tears. The first time was over our daughter Katie's diagnosis of oxalosis at birth.

Several hours later, Matt called to let me know Amy was resting well. When I left, he knew that spirit of confusion and defeat had to leave. He opened his Bible and began to read out loud to Amy and prayed. She then calmed down and fell asleep. I was finally able to fall asleep myself.

On Sunday, November 24th, Amy had been in the hospital three weeks. She was receiving dialysis six days a week. Since missing a day during the week, she had to have dialysis on that particular Sunday. We decided to go to church and then out to eat lunch together. None of us had eaten an actual sit down meal since Amy had been in the hospital.

Michael, Matt and I took Gabby and Jaelynn out to a restaurant. We had just sat down and started eating when suddenly I was struck in the top of the head. It almost knocked me out. In a few minutes, I regained enough of my senses to understand what caused my headache.

Beside our table had been standing a flag pole. On top of the pole, there was a brass eagle with its wings outstretched. For some unknown reason, the pole had fallen over at just the right angle to cause the tip of one of the wings to slam into the top of my head. It is a wonder the wing didn't split my head open.

"That thing just fell over for no reason," I heard the waitress say.

A large lump developed on the top of my head, and I was light headed and still seeing stars. (It is just not in cartoons that stars appear!) If the pole had fallen to either side of me, it would have hit Gabby or Jaelynn. It probably would have killed Jaelynn since she was only two years old and very tiny. Thank

God if it had to hit somebody, it was me. I have a very hard head, or so Michael tells me!

The waitress notified the restaurant manager, and somebody gave me an ice pack. The restaurant manager kept asking who had been messing with the pole because it just didn't fall over that easy. Nobody had touched it! We had all been sitting there quietly with the pole in the corner.

Michael took me to the hospital ER since the lump on my head was so large. At the hospital, an MRI was performed. Fortunately, I didn't have a cracked skull or any brain bleeds. I did have a concussion, and I was instructed to stay home and rest for a few days. For two days, I couldn't visit Amy and had to rely on Michael's reports. On the third day, he drove me to the hospital so I could see for myself that she was doing well.

I don't know why that pole fell and how it managed to be just the right distance away that it struck me with that brass wing tip right in the top of my head. No one else had an answer. Since there is a God, there must also be a satan. Satan probably thought he couldn't do much more to Amy; thus, he would try to get rid of me. I was the one taking care of Amy, getting her back on her feet. Satan couldn't handle that; he had failed! I was okay, and Amy was going to be fine too.

With Amy's improvement in early December, Matt knew he had to return to work. He needed the job. On January 1, he would receive medical insurance for himself, Amy and Joshua. Amy needed the insurance for her future medical bills. I was concerned how they would handle the stack of previous hospital bills. They would be expensive, especially since she had recently been to surgery three times and had spent days in

ICU. When Matt left his former job just before Amy became ill in August, he had been unable to keep the insurance due to it being too expensive.

While I was pondering what to do about helping them get the medical bills covered, I received a phone call from the social worker at the dialysis center. While working on the insurance coverage for Amy, she found that Amy could keep the insurance from Matt's former employer. Because she was on dialysis, the kidney foundation would pay the premiums. She was covered, including the present hospitalization. Praise God! This took a tremendous burden off them, all of us.

Amy was so confused from all the medications that we didn't want her staying alone. When Matt returned to Ohio, I stayed with her.

On Tuesday night, December 3, Amy went to sleep after receiving her bedtime medicine. I opened the cot in the far corner of the room so I could lie down. Soon, I was asleep. Suddenly, I felt somebody shaking me awake. Startled, I opened my eyes expecting to see Amy's nurse. I thought she wanted to ask me something, but no one was there. Looking over, I saw Amy sitting on the side of the bed at the foot. I jumped up and went to her.

"Amy, what are you doing?" I asked.

If she stood and tried to walk on her feet, she would have fallen. There was no telling what kind of damage she might have done to her feet, let alone possible other injuries.

"I need to go to the bathroom," she explained.

"Amy, did you forget about the catheter and your feet?"

"I forgot," she said. I helped her back up in the bed and then went back to the cot.

Who had shaken me awake? If I hadn't awakened, Amy would have fallen and been hurt. Was it Amy's guardian angel protecting her?

Plans began on December 4 for Amy's discharge. The unit manager wanted to send her to a nursing facility for care. Amy was very weak, unable to walk and had lost a lot of weight. She only weighed 88 pounds; her usual weight was 105 pounds. She required five hours of dialysis six days a week. Amy was not going to a nursing facility. I had always cared for her and would this time too. Anything that Amy needed, I would be able to do. She was not going to a facility surrounded by some people waiting to die. Amy was to be surrounded by life and love and that was at home!

Amy's lower feet and toes had turned black from the lack of circulation. Dr. Roese said several times they would have to be amputated. Amy would just look at him and say, "I'm keeping my toes."

Amy had surprised him several times, and he was willing to wait since there wasn't any infection in them. Just maybe, it would be like frost bite, and they would heal on their own.

A discussion was held with Amy's kidney doctor who ordered six days of dialysis while the dialysis centers only dialyzed patients three days a week. The only way Amy could get dialysis every day was to do home dialysis. A machine would be set up in our home and somebody needed to be trained to run it. I was nominated, but I didn't want to remove my daughter's blood from her body and then return it. There could be complications. I wanted a dialysis nurse, a trained expert.

If Amy's problems really were due to oxalosis, then we had to listen to the doctors concerning how much dialysis she needed. Amy thought about it and asked if I would do it. It was what she wanted, and I had to get comfortable with it quickly!

On December 14, Amy was discharged to our home. Counting the three days of ER visits, she had been in the hospital 40 days.

Chapter 19

The Struggle to Regain Strength

Amy couldn't walk and had to be lifted and carried. Our house sits on a hill, and the front door was not accessible. To get her into the house, we would drive the car up to the basement door. Then, she could be picked up and carried from the car to the basement stairs and carried up them. Michael and Matt could carry her, but we didn't know what to do when Matt wasn't there and Michael was at work. I couldn't carry her! The Hope Volunteer Fire Department came to our rescue. When I needed her up and down the stairs, I would call them. Some firefighters would arrive and provide much help. I don't know what we would have done without these wonderful men.

We needed a chairlift for the stairs. My niece, Lauren, started a Go Fund Me account on line. My brother, Daniel, also helped out financially. Soon we purchased a chairlift and had it installed about three weeks after Amy returned home.

Amy came home on Saturday. On Monday, we started our daily trek to the dialysis center for training. We had nine straight days of training with Christmas quickly approaching. I was completely exhausted and couldn't even think about Christmas, but I had two little girls and Joshua who expected Santa to arrive. It was three days before Christmas, and I didn't have the strength to dig out the Christmas tree. I had run into a department store one day to grab a few things and saw a display of a three foot tree with decorations, grabbed one and took it home. Michael placed it on a table. The kids now had a Christmas tree, a pitiful one, but they were happy. Fortunately,

I had bought Christmas presents months earlier so at least Santa could arrive!

On Christmas Eve, Amy's home dialysis machine arrived. I found it ironic that we were getting a dialysis machine for Christmas. The dialysis nurse scheduled training at home the day after Christmas.

Amy needed so much help when arriving home from the hospital. She had lost so much weight that she was skin and bones. She couldn't walk. We had to get a bedside commode and used a slide board to slide her from the bed to it or her wheelchair.

We moved a twin-size bed into my bedroom. The dialysis machine required water access and a sink for drainage; so, it was placed beside the master bathroom. Her bed was close to the machine, and I moved my bed to the corner. Even though her kidney wasn't working properly, it was still producing urine and her bladder was spastic, requiring her to get up multiple times during the night. Poor Michael was sent to the upstairs guest bedroom to sleep. All his stuff went with him to make room for all the medical supplies.

After two more weeks of home training, the dialysis center pronounced us ready for solo runs. Thank God for Jill Ross, our dialysis nurse. I suspect I drove her crazy calling every day with a question about something that was going wrong. She was always so pleasant and made sure I had all her phone numbers if needing her expertise.

Amy had to run five hours for each treatment. The doctor wanted her to have them six days a week because of the oxalate. Amy refused to have one on Saturday. The weekends were the only time for her family! She didn't want to spend the day on dialysis instead of spending time with Matt and Joshua. The doctor stated it was her decision. I also felt it was important for Amy to be with them. Saturday was scratched off the schedule!

A few days after getting discharged from the hospital, Amy was scheduled to start going to the Columbus Wound Center, a wonderful facility, for treatment of her feet. Her feet and toes had become black and hard. At her first appointment, she had to see a doctor never seen before. When the bandages were removed, I thought the doctor was going to pass out.

"Has anyone seen your feet since they turned black?" she asked Amy.

"Yes," Amy replied.

"Well, you need to see your vascular surgeon today. I want him to look at this."

She called Dr. Roese's office and came back into the room to say we were to go directly to his office. One of the surgeons would see her when we arrived.

I took Amy back out to the car and drove to their office. Back into the wheelchair, we hurried into the office where she was taken to an exam room. Dr. Christy arrived and looked at her feet. Her feet looked exactly like he had anticipated. He was still hoping they would not need to be amputated completely but cautioned Amy she would likely lose her toes.

"I'm keeping my toes," she informed him.

"I hope so," he answered.

She was scheduled every week to see a doctor at the Columbus Wound Center. The following week, she met the foot surgeon, Dr. Hladik. He said, "Your feet are mummified."

"I don't want to lose my feet," she told him.

He examined her feet. Over the next few weeks, he would remove the blackened tissue a little at a time. If there were good tissue under it, he would continue to do so; if he found dead tissue under the black skin, then it would be time to amputate. Amy agreed to the plan and the procedure would start the following week.

By late February, I was even more exhausted than previously. I was running her for five hours of dialysis, but it took much longer for me. I had to set up the machine prior to the treatment and then tear it down and clean it; I had to keep up an inventory of the supplies we needed and order supplies from the dialysis center, some from the dialysis company and some from the company that provided the bags of saline. I had to make sure medicines were ordered and picked up and schedule all her appointments.

Without sleep, I do not function well. Amy was getting me up several times a night. As soon as I was asleep, Amy would need me. Finally, Amy regained some strength and figured out that she could slide out of bed on her knees and crawl to the bathroom without awakening me. Then, she would crawl back. Her toes were as hard as a hard plastic doll. As she crawled, I could hear her toes tap, tapping on the tile floor. As I listened to that tap, tapping, the sound would break my heart. I would cry silently so she couldn't hear.

I questioned God. Amy had been through so much in her life. Why did she have to endure all these trials? He had brought her through many things; He would this too; but, I hated to see her suffer.

Toward the end of February, Michael became ill with a stomach virus. He had a fever, vomiting and diarrhea. I depended on him a lot! He took care of the girls and Joshua so I could care for Amy. When he was at work, Katie would come over and watch the kids. Two days later, Amy woke up with the same symptoms. She also had elevated blood pressure and chest pain. I took her to the emergency room, and she was admitted.

The hospital doctor caring for her asked to discuss her case out in the hall. She stressed that Amy's feet were making her ill, and they needed to be amputated.

"I need you to convince Amy to have her feet amputated."

"I'm sorry; I can't do that. It is Amy's decision. Besides, I think she has the same stomach virus my husband is fighting. That is what is making her sick."

"No, her feet are making her ill. She needs them amputated."

I knew in my heart that wasn't the case, that it was a virus. I repeated, "She has the same virus as my husband. Amy may need to have her feet amputated, but not now. It will be Amy's decision if reaching that point."

The doctor was obviously upset with my answer.

"Fine. We will call it a stomach virus!"

She turned and walked away. I went across the hall and entered a bathroom. Why, oh why am I forced to take strong stands about Amy's care? Why can't they see things the way they were?

Eventually, I calmed myself and I reentered Amy's room. A different doctor was talking with Amy suggesting she might have a heart blockage, probably caused by the same spasms that had affected her legs. After he left, Amy was very upset. We were not going to believe it. Besides, God would correct it! The following day, another doctor informed us she didn't have a blockage. The EKG they did was normal!

That night, Dr. Hladik saw Amy. If she continued to have an elevated temperature, he would need to amputate her feet. I think the other doctor was applying some pressure to proceed with the surgery. Amy told him okay, but she would not have a fever any longer. He advised it might be difficult for her to control.

Amy's temp remained normal the rest of the night and remained normal the following morning when he returned. Dr. Hladik assured her he wouldn't amputate and would resume their previous plan as promised. She was discharged later that day.

So, we continued our dialysis routine at home and went to the Columbus Wound Center on Fridays. Dr. Hladik started removing the blackened skin from her feet. Underneath, he found good live tissue. The first time he found it, he was joyful. We were happy; Amy's feet were coming back! She kept saying she could feel her toes, that they felt like they were trapped inside a concrete shoe.

Amy was still gaining strength and was crawling around the house to get to her destinations rather than depending on me and the wheelchair. I was doing dressing changes on her feet twice a day, once in the morning while she was on dialysis and then in the evening.

Dialysis was going fairly well, but she would have episodes of low blood pressure. I would seldom have to take fluid off her; if I did, then her blood pressure would drop even lower. One day during dialysis, Amy suddenly didn't feel right and appeared to pass out. Her eyes became set. Quickly, I took her blood pressure. It had dropped to 30/10! I thought she was going to die and yelled for Michael while opening the saline line and running fluid into her. Her blood pressure came up to 60/30, and her eyes looked a little better. I proceeded to run saline in while Michael paced the floor.

"Do you want me to call an ambulance?" he asked.

By then, her blood pressure was still climbing, and she was starting to respond. Finally, she was normal but couldn't recall anything other than feeling dizzy. She was better, but I was shaking like a leaf. What if she would die during one of these episodes?

At the end of February, Amy began to complain of headaches at the base of her skull. When bending her head forward, she would become light headed. I wondered if it had something to do with the Chiari malformation that was diagnosed when she was an infant. This malformation was an opening in the base of the skull that would let the brain stem fall through. It had been followed over the years but had never caused a problem.

I thought it was best if we checked with her doctor about the symptoms. He ordered an MRI. On February 28th, she went for the exam. That evening, someone called Amy from the hospital and reported the MRI was normal. The malformation was apparently no longer there. The person didn't know how because they just didn't disappear, but it was gone! We figured this was a miracle from God, and it helped to build our faith higher for Amy's complete healing. The headaches and dizziness disappeared too.

We continued to believe that Amy's feet would completely heal even though my eyes told me something different. Her right foot began to shrivel, and I was afraid it might actually break off. I kept my fears to myself and persisted in praising God for the healing of her feet.

In mid-April during Amy's wound center visit, Dr. Hladik removed some more black skin and did not find good tissue. He found what he described as mush. The healing had ended.

"It is time Amy; it has stopped healing."

Tearfully she accepted what she had battled so long. He scheduled surgery for April 22. I had to hold back my tears. On the way home, we both cried.

Dr. Hladik came in to see her after admission. He looked at her feet and ordered total bedrest. He was afraid her right foot was literally going to fall off. We talked. He would only remove what was absolutely necessary to preserve as much of her feet as possible, especially the heels so it would be easier for her to learn to walk again.

Matt arrived and spent the night with her. The next morning, she was taken to surgery. Our pastors arrived to pray with her and to sit with us during the surgery. While we waited, I prayed the doctor would not have to remove much.

When the surgery was over, we were taken to the consultation room to speak with Dr. Hladik. He removed half of Amy's left foot. The right foot had been in worse condition, and he removed the entire foot but saved the heel. It seemed so strange. The left foot had been in the worse condition when she had the circulation loss. Why was it the opposite now?

I felt so heartbroken for Amy and so confused. We had been so sure God would heal her feet. I wasn't sure how I would explain to Gabby and Jaelynn why God didn't heal her; I couldn't even comprehend it myself.

Once Amy was taken from recovery to her room, we were allowed to see her. She had huge dressings on her feet, but I could tell they were missing. I was so sad and broke down crying. Pastor Dona hugged me, but I could feel nothing but heartbreak for what Amy was going through.

She only remained in the hospital four days before being released to our home. Matt was really good about keeping Amy's spirits up and talking with her about keeping her faith. Losing her feet was not what we wanted and had believed would happen, but she could have lost her legs or even her life. She was doing better than everyone thought. We just needed to get her healed, get her prosthetics and back to walking.

Amy seemed to accept the way things were. She went back to reading her Bible and listening to her healing CDs. I couldn't really tell how she felt, but I was physically, emotionally and spiritually exhausted. Gabby and Jaelynn never asked why God didn't heal Amy, so I was spared that conversation. I didn't know how to answer such a question anyway.

Chapter 20

The Daily Routine Continues

In early May, Katie told us she was pregnant, at last a little joy in our lives-another grandchild! She had two boys, so maybe this one would be our first granddaughter. We didn't know if Amy would be happy or if the news would depress her. I knew Amy wanted more children. It seemed unlikely to ever happen.

Amy was not feeling well, frequently having fevers. Finally, a diagnosis was obtained. She had an infection in her dialysis catheter. She was taken to surgery and the catheter replaced.

On June 3rd after Amy had gone to bed, she awakened me. Her stomach was hurting badly. She also felt nauseated. I got out of bed to get a pan knowing she would vomit since it was at least an every other day occurrence being on dialysis. Amy kept moaning. Her stomach really hurt a lot. Suddenly, she vomited. Looking at the contents in the pan, I knew it contained blood.

We were going to ER once again. I got dressed quickly. All she could do was moan, clutch her stomach and vomit repeatedly. I went to the foot of the stairs and yelled for Michael. While he was getting dressed, I managed to get Amy into her wheelchair and to the chairlift. She was so weak I couldn't get her into the seat of the chairlift. I thought she was going to pass out, and I took her to the sofa. Michael helped me lay her down. She was so pale, so sick. It would be impossible to get her into the car!

"Call an ambulance now," I told Michael.

Within minutes, a sheriff's deputy arrived. He let the ambulance driver know exactly the location of our house and how to get up our long drive. It seemed to take a long time for the ambulance to arrive, but I'm sure it wasn't really. The paramedics assessed her, started an IV, put her on a stretcher and then into the ambulance. Michael stayed with the kids while I followed the ambulance.

Once at the hospital, it was confirmed Amy was vomiting blood. She was admitted. Early in the morning, she was taken to surgery for a scope of her stomach. A bleeding ulcer was found, and she was put on medication.

After Amy was returned to her room, I received a call from Katie. She was crying. Her baby didn't have a heartbeat during an ultrasound. I was starting to wonder how much more stress our family could possibly handle.

She was only eight weeks pregnant, but it was still devastating. This was the second time she had lost a baby. The first time was when Jayden was four years old; that baby also suddenly didn't have a heartbeat. The doctor delayed almost two weeks before doing a D&C. The wait had been difficult for Katie; thus, this particular surgery was scheduled for the next day.

Katie arrived at the hospital. I met her and Chris at the entrance and walked with her to surgery admitting. I had decided not to tell Amy until she was home. She had enough of her own problems! Katie had the procedure, did well and Chris took her home. I went back to Amy's room. She had been in dialysis while Katie had been in surgery.

144

Amy was in the hospital for a week before being discharged. While in the hospital, the staff removed a lot of fluid from her during dialysis. We kept telling them not to, that she didn't need fluid removed because her kidney was still producing urine. Somehow, our communication was not forwarded to the proper person. When she was discharged, her weight was down four pounds; her blood pressure was low; she felt ill and looked very ill. I knew she needed out of the hospital. It would be better for her to be dialyzed at home so I could control how much fluid was removed. Even though she was still sick when they discharged her, I didn't object. I just took her home.

The next morning when it was time for dialysis, Amy was feeling even worse. I hooked her up, but her blood pressure, which was low, dropped even more. She started having chest pains and began vomiting. I took her back off and called her dialysis nurse to let her know I couldn't run Amy because she was so dry. She instructed me to have her drink chicken broth. The sodium would cause fluid to remain in her tissues.

I explained to Amy she needed to drink it, or she would be back in the hospital. I gave her medicine for her nausea. As she drank the broth over the next few hours, I could see an improvement. The next day, she was able to tolerate dialysis.

Two months after the stomach bleed, the gastroenterologist performed another scope on Amy's stomach to check on the ulcer. He found the ulcer had healed so well he couldn't even tell where it had been.

A few months after her amputations, Dr. Hladik decided to have Amy take treatments in a hyperbaric oxygen chamber. He felt this would help heal her feet. She would need to go every day after dialysis.

We were now doing dialysis Monday through Friday from 8 a.m. until 1 p.m. Treatments in the chamber were every day from 3 p.m. until about 4:30. At that time, she also had another infection in her dialysis catheter and had to go to the hospital for IV antibiotics three times a week. She had to be there at 5 p.m.

We didn't know how we were going to get this accomplished. Katie watched the kids during the day when Michael had to work, but she had to be home by 3:00 when Jayden arrived from school. Jaelynn could go with us to the appointments. She was three years old and listened. Joshua, on the other hand, was not yet two. It would be too difficult to get Amy to the appointments and handle both Jaelynn and Joshua while loading and unloading Amy from her wheelchair.

After some discussion, Amy made the decision to send Joshua back to Ohio with Matt. Matt's parents could help care for him. I hated to see Amy send her son away, but I also knew she didn't feel well enough to care for him. It took some of the responsibility off Michael and me. I had Gabby take the school bus with Jayden to his parents' house, and she would stay with Katie until Michael or I could pick her up.

For the next three months, I would get up at 6 a.m. and get the dialysis machine ready. Then, I would get the girls up and ready for the day. I would put Amy on dialysis by 7:30. Michael would take Gabby to school before he went to work.

While I ran Amy on dialysis, Jaelynn would watch television or play in her room. I would clean the kitchen and Jaelynn would come into the bedroom for preschool. Often, I would have to stop and deal with the alarms on the machine, Amy becoming ill or her blood pressure dropping. Every 30 minutes, I would have to do her vital signs and check pressures on the machine and record them. If alarms went off, I had to determine what was causing it such as blood clots, air in the lines or something else and fix the problem.

She was supposed to run for five hours, but the machine didn't seem to understand and would run for an additional 15-20 minutes. Some days, I really needed that extra few minutes for something else! By the time the treatment was over and I had gotten Amy off, the machine tore down and scrubbed with bleach, it would be about 1:30. I would get myself, Amy and Jaelynn ready and be at the wound center by 3:00. After dropping Amy off, Jaelynn and I would run errands and return to pick Amy up by 4:30. Then, we would go to the hospital for her IV antibiotics which would take until 7:00. Thankfully, she only had to have a couple of weeks of IV antibiotics two different times during the three months she was going to the chamber!

When arriving back home, I would be so tired. If Michael wasn't home to cook supper, I would pick up fast food from a restaurant drive through for the girls. They also ate a lot of pizza rolls during those weeks.

Dr. Hladik wanted to do skin grafts to her feet. When applying to Amy's insurance company, they turned the procedure down. Dr. Hladik felt the grafts were what Amy needed, but he would try to figure something else out.

147

Since her insurance wouldn't pay for skin grafts, Dr. Hladik was going to put a different type of graft on Amy's right foot which was having problems healing. On October 12, he took her to surgery. Afterwards, he came out and said he had put a skin graft on Amy's right foot. There had been enough left over to put one also on her left foot. I didn't ask how he had accomplished this since the insurance company had refused to pay for the procedure. Some things are just better left unasked!

Amy came out of surgery with large bandages on both feet. She looked as if her feet had been stuck into basketballs.

In November, Amy started crying and tossing about in her sleep causing me to wake up. I would wake her up to ask if she was in pain, which she would deny. After many nights of this behavior, she opened up about what was bothering her. She was having dreams of Dr. Brown molesting her. These thoughts had not bothered her for years, and we didn't know why she was having these dreams again. I told her to tell the dreams to stop and to think good thoughts before going to sleep. We both lie back down. Amy was dealing with enough physically; she certainly didn't need to be tormented emotionally. I had had it with all these problems.

"You are to stop bothering Amy. Do not touch her ever again in the name of Jesus."

We both fell asleep. Before long, I was suddenly waking up. Somebody was touching me, actually molesting me! I opened my eyes. Standing over me was a very scary looking man. I had never seen a demon before, not sure I believed in them. Pastor Mark had talked about them. Now, what was standing over me was surely a demon. I raised my hand and pointed to it.

"You cannot touch Amy. You cannot touch me or anyone else in this house. I order you out of my house and our lives in the name of Jesus." Suddenly, it was gone.

"And don't come back," I yelled.

That was strange, I thought. The demon must have decided it would try to drive me crazy since it couldn't bother Amy. I knew it would not be back. Amy has not been bothered since that night, and the terrible dreams have stopped.

Chapter 21

Life Continues

2015 rolled in with not much changing. We continued doing dialysis five hours a day. I continued changing Amy's stump dressings two times a day, and she continued going to the Columbus Wound Center every Friday. She was no longer taking treatments in the hyperbaric chamber. Twice a month she went to the dialysis clinic, once to see the kidney doctor and once for clinic with the dialysis nurse.

Nothing changed with her stumps. The left was healing slowly, but the right one seemed at a standstill. Dr. Hladik would change her treatments every so often.

The kidney doctor began to talk about a transplant. She was remarkedly healthy despite everything, and he felt we needed to pursue it. Every doctor Amy saw had a different opinion. Most thought it would be better if receiving a new liver and kidney. Having a liver transplant would cure the oxalosis. Other doctors thought, since she did well for 27 years, maybe another kidney was all she needed. We didn't want her to have a liver transplant if it wasn't necessary. That seemed so drastic, like replacing one set of problems for a different set of problems.

Amy was given an appointment at Indiana University Hospital to see Dr. Sharon Moe. She was a nephrologist specializing in oxalate disease. On January 29th, Amy, Katie and I went to the appointment. Katie wanted to donate a kidney to her sister. At the appointment, Dr. Moe went over Amy's history. There were several different types of oxalosis. If Amy actually had primary oxalosis, it was unlikely that she could have kept a transplanted kidney for 27 years. That just wasn't feasible. Blood was drawn from Amy and from Katie and me. Dr. Moe wanted to see what type of defective gene I carried that Amy had inherited and if Katie also had inherited it. The blood had to be sent to the Mayo Clinic in Minnesota; so, it would take weeks to get the results. Back home we went to wait for the results.

We hoped and prayed the results would prove Amy did not have primary oxalosis. If she didn't, she would not need a liver transplant. We also could stop the five hour a day dialysis and just do three hours like other kidney failure patients. Three hour runs would help with my chronic exhaustion.

While we waited, Amy continued to see Dr. Hladik weekly for her stumps. He decided to have an MRI done to her right ankle and leg to see if there was a problem with the bone such as infection or dead bone.

On March 26th, we returned to see Dr. Moe for the results of the genetic tests. We prayed and believed we would get good results. Our prayers seemed to be in vain. When Dr. Moe came in, the news was not what we wanted to hear. The results diagnosed Amy as having primary oxalosis. She had two different genes which resulted in the disease, one from me and the other from Michael. Katie also had the gene from her father but had received a normal gene from me. So, she did not have the disease but is a carrier.

Dr. Moe very carefully explained all the results and then stated that Amy would need a liver transplant to cure the disease. She also believed that Amy needed dialysis seven days a week but felt three hour treatments were long enough to remove the oxalate from her blood. Getting the dialysis treatments changed from five hours to three hours was the only positive thing to come from the meeting. Amy and I once again were depressed by terrible information, and Amy cried all the way back to the car. This was another mountain we seemed to be struggling through without God's help. Where was He in all this? Amy still had oxalosis, and her stumps were not healing, even after receiving the skin grafts.

Amy did not want dialysis seven days a week. She wanted the weekend for Matt and Joshua, the only normal things that she seemed to have left. We talked all the way home, and I finally persuaded her to do six days a week.

"We can do the three hours early on Saturday morning, and you will have the rest of the day to spend with them and all day Sunday."

We still felt that if she had stayed healthy for 27 years living with oxalosis that surely she could have a good life again with just another kidney transplant.

The following day, Amy had another appointment with Dr. Hladik to find out the results of the MRI. Once more, we received horrible news. There was infection in the bone, and part of it was dead. She would need her right leg amputated below the knee. Amy cried when hearing the news. It was all I could do to hold myself together for her. Dr. Hladik stressed the stump would not heal until more was amputated. Once it was amputated, it would heal. She would be walking sooner. Amy reluctantly agreed to the surgery, and Dr. Hladik would schedule it with Dr. Roese.

Back in the car, Amy and I both cried. I was so sad she had to go through so many trials. Two days in a row, we had received devastating news. I couldn't take much more myself, and I was frightened for Amy's disposition. I was afraid she would just give up.

On April 27th, Amy was admitted to the hospital for more surgery. It had been a year since her foot amputations. I asked Dr. Roese if the part of her leg amputated could be tested to determine how much oxalate was in the blood vessels and in the tissue of her leg. No one still had a definite reason for the circulation problems. They just theorized it was due to oxalate saturation. He would arrange with the pathology lab to test it.

Amy returned from surgery minus her right lower leg. Everyone attempted to keep her spirits up. We all talked about how it would heal faster and how she would be able to get her prosthetics sooner. Amy didn't talk much about the surgery. I knew this was a hurdle we needed to get through, but how were we to get her out of kidney failure?

We kept praying and praising God for healing her kidney. Every day, Amy and I would get up and thank Him for this day being the last day she would need dialysis. The next day, we would get up and climb the same mountain. I would tell God that we wanted a miracle and that we needed it now, always sure of it.

Several days after the surgery, Dr. Roese gave us the report from the pathology lab. The results showed that the vessels in the amputated leg were full of oxalate crystal as was the tissue, another devastating blow!

Since Amy now had to learn to move about without her lower leg, she was transferred to the hospital's rehab unit about four days after the surgery. She received dialysis every morning at the hospital followed by physical and occupational therapies the rest of the day. Matt returned to Ohio. The girls and I would go around dinnertime every day and visit as she ate. We would stay until it was her bedtime.

After two weeks in rehab, Amy was discharged. We resumed our prior schedule of dialysis every morning. During dialysis, she didn't pay any attention to the Christian shows I would turn to on the television. All she did was sleep while denying she was in pain. After dialysis, I would transfer Amy from bed to her wheelchair and take her to the living room. If she didn't have an appointment that day, I would attempt to get her to read or listen to one of her CDs. She would refuse. If I turned on the television, she would seemingly look through it. She wouldn't choose anything to watch. She didn't talk unless she had to answer my questions. She made no attempts to move her wheelchair herself. She stayed right where I left her. Amy didn't do anything but sit and stare into space!

I didn't know what to do to help; I didn't even know what to pray for any more. One day, I fought with the dialysis machine which kept alarming. As Amy stared into the ceiling unconcerned as to the reason for the alarms, I found myself leaning against the wall and banging my head, teetering on the edge myself. All I could do was cry and say the only thing I knew to say, "Jesus, Jesus, Jesus." We both needed help or neither one of us would get through this challenging period.

I picked up my phone, called Amy's doctor and made an appointment. I knew Amy had to get out of the mood she was in, and I requested an antidepressant. The doctor wrote a prescription.

Two weeks after starting the medicine, I began to see a change in Amy. She started talking and wheeling herself around in her wheelchair. Everywhere I went, she followed me! With Amy's spirits lifted, I began to feel better myself. I was gaining a little more energy for our next struggle.

Chapter 22

Making a Decision

In June, Amy's kidney doctor sent a referral to Indiana University Medical Center for an evaluation for a kidney transplant. We went for an appointment with a nephrologist. Amy and I discussed her history and how her transplanted kidney had lasted 27 years. He agreed that another kidney transplant would likely do just as well. He said he would start the process to put her on the transplant list. If Katie wanted to donate a kidney, then they would also start that process.

We were excited. Somebody finally agreed that a liver transplant wasn't necessary. We certainly didn't want it. Her liver worked well except for missing the enzyme that broke down oxalate. She had lived all her life with oxalosis, and we really felt her circulation problems were due to drugs. If it was the oxalate, why wasn't she still having problems? We were also concerned about the risks with two transplants, kidney and liver.

On June 26th, we received a call from the transplant coordinator that Amy had been placed on the kidney transplant list. They still wanted her to see a liver doctor for consultation. On July 15, the coordinator called back. The doctors had changed their minds. They refused to do just a kidney transplant. They would only do a liver and kidney transplant feeling the oxalosis was too severe and another kidney transplant would fail. They made an appointment for Amy to see one of their liver doctors.

We couldn't figure out why they had changed their minds. We were upset, but there was no way to reverse the decision. Amy had to make the call. If she refused a liver transplant, we would have to find another transplant center. It was not very likely another center would do just a kidney either.

Over the next few weeks, Amy watched videos of healing. For some reason, she started seeing stories about people who had received liver transplants. They all shared how God had protected them through the transplant and how they were doing really well afterwards.

In a few days, Amy chose to have a liver transplant. She felt at peace about it. On August 10, 2015, Amy and I went to IU to see the liver doctor. Based on the genetic tests and the crystals found in her vessels, she really needed the liver and kidney transplant. He would start the process to put her on the transplant list, and she probably would have about a four month wait based on previous transplants at the center.

During the next two months, Amy had to undergo many medical tests to prove she was healthy enough for both transplants. She passed all the tests!

The transplant coordinator called us on December 2nd to tell us the transplant board had approved her for the liver and kidney transplant. Next, the hospital had to apply for financial approval from Amy's insurance. She indicated it would take about a week.

The next day, the coordinator called to tell us the insurance company had approved the transplants. We were shocked to get the approval back so quickly!

Amy's right stump had healed, and she had received a temporary prosthetic for that leg. The transplant team wanted Amy walking by the time she received her transplants. Walking would help with recovery. Dr. Hladik ordered a special boot for her left foot that she could walk on but that would also promote healing.

A few days after getting the boot, we stopped at a convenience store to get drinks. I asked Amy if she wanted to go in. Amy had not been in a convenience store for over two years! It had just been too inconvenient to get the wheelchair out of the trunk and get her in it to just run in for a few minutes.

"Do you think I can?" she asked

"Amy, you can do anything you want. You can walk now."

"Yes, I want to go in," she replied with a big smile.

I helped her out of the car, gave her the walker and together we entered. She walked about the store and looked all around. We returned to the car, and I asked her how that had felt.

"Good. It's been a long time," she answered, still smiling from ear to ear.

We don't realize how little tiny things can mean so much to us until we can no longer do them. I can no longer jump out of my car and run into a store without being thankful.

On December 10th, 2015, we received the call informing us that Amy had been placed on the transplant list. We were told to always answer the phone when it rang, even if not recognizing the number. My phone was first on the list. Amy's was next, but she did not always answer it. Many times she was asleep, on dialysis, at a doctor's appointment or physical therapy. Matt's phone was third on the list, but he could not always answer it while at work. My phone stayed with me constantly. Even at church, I had my phone on vibrate in my hand. When we received that call, we were not going to miss it!

Close to Christmas, Amy's foot wound seemed to have stopped healing, and Dr. Hladik requested she stay off it for a few weeks to help with the healing. She had to go back to her wheelchair. Amy was determined to take Joshua to visit Santa even if it meant going in a wheelchair. So, off to the mall they went.

As they waited in line, Joshua told Amy and Matt what toys he was going to ask Santa to bring. When it was finally Joshua's turn, Santa asked him what he wanted for Christmas. Joshua looked at Santa and didn't ask for any of the toys. Instead, he said "I want my mommy well, so she can come home."

Santa looked over at Amy waiting in her wheelchair and motioned for her and Matt to approach him. He inquired of them about Amy's condition. After hearing the brief version of the story, he turned back to Joshua.

"Joshua, I can't make your mommy well, but there is someone who can. That is Jesus. Do you believe that?" Joshua nodded his head.

Santa turned back to Amy and asked if he could pray for her. There in the mall with the crowd waiting, Santa bowed his head and prayed for Amy's healing.

It was an amazing scene. Santa was making a prayer request on behalf of a little boy for a gift that Santa could not provide, a gift of a healthy mommy who could return home to her son.

Santa said he would be there the following Christmas, and Amy promised to return and let him know how she was doing.

A few weeks later, Amy woke with ear pain. I was afraid she might have an infection and took her to the doctor. Amy had to be healthy when receiving the call for her transplants. We could not take any chances! She didn't have an infection but had what appeared to be a tiny fluid-filled cyst. The doctor lanced and drained it.

The next day, Amy woke up with her nose swollen and red. Over the next three days, her nose continued to swell and be very painful. Another doctor's appointment and a trip to ER didn't cure it or even give us a diagnosis.

Finally, on January 4th, the transplant coordinator asked me to take her to an IU hospital in Indianapolis. There, she was diagnosed with MRSA, and an ENT doctor drained a large cyst in her nasal cavity. Amy was admitted and given strong IV antibiotics. She stayed in the hospital three days and then was sent home with a supply of antibiotics.

Because she was on the transplant waiting list, she had lab work done every week. The transplant team needed the results to see how Amy was doing and to match her with a donor when they received organs. On February 29ᵗʰ, 2016, we were making one of our weekly treks to the hospital. Amy had done well that day on dialysis. She had eaten lunch, gotten dressed and then walked to the car. We talked on the way to the hospital.

As I pulled the car into a parking spot, Amy suddenly said, "Something's wrong, Mom; I don't feel right."

I looked over at her, and she fell forward as if she had passed out.

"Amy," I called and touched her shoulder. She didn't respond. I didn't know what could be wrong. She had been fine. I knew what I had to do, and I put my hands on her.

"Lord, whatever it is, fix it," I prayed.

Suddenly, Amy sat up. I was somewhat relieved but still very concerned. "Amy, what happened?" I asked.

"I don't know; I just suddenly felt weird and dizzy. Now, I have chest pain and feel light headed."

I decided to take her to the ER and backed the car out and drove to the entrance. A valet met me and parked the car while I put Amy in a wheelchair and took her in.

Going into the ER, I saw the place was crowded but was hoping they could make Amy a priority. After registering Amy at the desk, we waited with others but fortunately not long. Somebody called Amy's name, and they took her history and vital signs. She was then placed in an exam room. A doctor arrived and ordered an EKG and other tests. An IV was started in her arm, and she was given pain medications.

We were there a couple of hours before receiving the test results. Amy's EKG was normal. She hadn't had a heart attack! All her blood work was okay for a kidney failure patient, and a chest x-ray was also normal. The doctor didn't know why she had passed out, but she apparently no longer had the problem. We didn't know but believed God had intervened and fixed it.

Amy was constantly bombarded by some problem. The following week, she would wake up in the mornings with the left side of her face swollen. After dialysis and as the day progressed, the swelling would diminish some. Her kidney doctor finally saw the swelling. He believed she might have a clot in the blood vessel where the dialysis catheter was placed. There wasn't anything that could be done about it. We just needed to watch it. This didn't sound good to me. I thought it sounded like a ticking time bomb, something that could cause serious problems.

We knew all these problems that kept cropping up had to stop. On Sunday, Amy had Pastor Mark pray about the swelling. The next morning, she woke up with it gone for the first time in a week!

Chapter 23

A Double Transplant

Once Amy had been placed on the transplant list, a new set of worries kept trying to invade my head. We had to be ready the minute we received the call. The Transplant Center was an hour away.

What if the call came at bedtime? I was so exhausted when the day was over, I would literally fall into bed sometimes with my clothes still on. If the call came during the night, how was I to have the strength to get Amy to the hospital and deal with her going into surgery?

It would take Matt at least two hours to get to the hospital from Ohio. Katie had started a job and would not be available to come quickly to stay with Gabby and Jaelynn. Michael would want to be at the hospital too; so, he couldn't stay with the kids. Everybody we knew worked and had their own responsibilities. How were we going to get help? It would be up to me to get Amy there!

I worried and stewed about these problems for days. I kept coming up with plans that probably would not work. Finally, one day as I prayed, I heard God say, "Would you let Me handle it?"

I turned it over to Him and promised to stop worrying about it. Sometimes it is hard to stop worrying about things when I want them to develop a certain way, and they don't.

Not too long after, Katie called. She had quit her job feeling she needed to be at home with her boys and wanting to be available when we received the call.

March 10th started out like every other day. I had Amy on dialysis by 8:00 a.m. As typical, I was hooking her up and thanking God for this being the last day she would need dialysis. I started questioning if I really had the faith needed. However, the Bible says to keep asking and believing, and I didn't know anything else to do.

At 11:00, my phone rang. When I picked it up, I saw it was the transplant office which wasn't unusual. Now and then, the coordinator would call to share information or ask questions. As I looked at the number, I just knew this was the call! When answering, the coordinator asked how Amy was doing. After telling her Amy was well and sleeping, she told me they had a possible liver and kidney. Since Amy was due to come off dialysis in 30 minutes, I was to finish the treatment and then take her to the hospital. I knew that getting her off, helping her get ready and then driving there would take at least till 1:30. According to the coordinator, our timing would be perfect.

The timing of this call was perfect too. I wasn't totally exhausted. Amy was dialyzed and ready for it. She already had an appointment in Indianapolis for 2:00; so, I had everything ready for that appointment as soon as she got off dialysis. Michael was home from work that day and had just left to make a quick run to a local store.

After we hung up, I talked with God. "Okay, we have believed you would heal Amy of the oxalosis and kidney failure.

You can still heal her right up to the moment we get there. I didn't want her to go through a liver and another kidney transplant. If this is the way it is to go, then I trust you. I know it will be perfect, and I thank you!"

I woke Amy and told her we were going to the hospital for new organs instead of the appointment for her prosthesis. She looked happy and called Matt to let him know.

We had already made plans for Katie to pick Jaelynn up at 12:00 from preschool and come to our house. Katie was going with us to the appointment. Then she, Amy and I were planning on spending some time together shopping while Michael kept the girls and Katie's boys.

Michael came home from the store and was given the news. Once Katie arrived with Jaelynn and Charlie, we all decided that Katie should go with us to the hospital. It would be quite a while before we knew if the liver and kidney was compatible with Amy. Michael does not do well with waiting. He would stay home with the kids until we knew if the surgery was definitely a go. Then, I would call him, and he would head to the hospital. My brother, Daniel, also happened to be off work that day. He would stay with the kids during the surgery until one of us could return home. The entire process could not have worked out better.

"Thank you God for handling it," I repeated over and over.

When we arrived at the hospital, Amy was directed to the Transplant Outpatient Unit. There, we waited while tests were performed on Amy and the donor organs. We arrived at 1:30, but we were told even if the surgery was performed that it wouldn't happen until late that evening. Blood was drawn from Amy and other procedures were performed. We watched as patients arrived to possibly receive transplants. Several of them left. For some reason, they weren't getting a transplant. We knew Amy could also be sent home but somehow knew this was Amy's day. Amy would be well today!

At 7:00, a transplant surgeon arrived and told us the organs were very healthy. He was quite sure Amy would get them. It would be another hour or so until we received the official go. First, Amy would receive the liver transplant. She would remain on continuous dialysis for three days and would then return to surgery for the kidney transplant. The surgeons had found patients did better with a three-day wait between the surgeries. She would then stay on dialysis for a while until the new kidney was functioning well hoping to remove as much oxalate as possible from her blood so as to protect it.

I called Michael and let him know that we had received an unofficial go. He would head to the hospital after calling Pastor Mark. At 7:45, the nurse came in to tell us Amy was heading to surgery in 10 minutes. Matt was there, and his parents had just walked in the door. The family gathered around Amy asking God for His blessing and to look over Amy and the surgeons.

The staff arrived to transport Amy to surgery. We were allowed to walk to the surgery doors with her, where we gave her hugs and kisses and assured her everything would go great. Amy looked happy and at peace. It is difficult to describe all the emotions as we watched her being wheeled away.

We were directed to the waiting area and would receive updates on a phone in the room. We were the only family there. Michal didn't arrive until after the surgery had started, and our pastors arrived a short time afterward.

I tried not to think about what was actually happening to Amy. The doctors were removing my daughter's liver, a liver that was just missing that darn enzyme that broke down oxalate. I couldn't dwell on that; I needed to concentrate on the fact that Amy would no longer have oxalosis. She would not have oxalate crystals building up in her bones, eyes, blood vessels and who knew where else. This was her opportunity to be free of a terrible disease.

A couple of hours into surgery, we received a call telling us the doctors had removed her liver and were starting to stitch in the new one. The nurse said that Amy was doing well.

The surgery lasted about six hours. We spent the time visiting with our pastors and some family friends who had arrived. When the surgery was over, about 2 a.m., the surgeon came out and reported Amy was doing well. The liver was working, and he expected everything to proceed well.

The liver tests from Friday through Sunday showed the liver was functioning perfectly. Once Amy was back in her room and was allowed to start taking liquids by mouth, she surprised us all by requesting a grape popsicle. The first popsicle she bit into shocked Matt and me. We were standing beside her bed and watching. Amy had never eaten popsicles in her life! She had been offered them after her many surgeries but always refused them. Her teeth were also sensitive to cold, but she ate the popsicle as it were the tastiest thing ever. It didn't even bother her teeth. Matt and I would watch her eat one after the other and marvel at this sudden change.

On Sunday morning at 8 a.m., Amy was taken back to surgery for the kidney transplant. The kidney surgeon explained that Amy had very high antibodies against the organ. He felt we needed to do everything possible to prevent possible rejection. Therefore, he wanted to use the best antirejection drugs available. These were the drugs we felt had caused terrible circulation in her legs. He promised if Amy had any problems after starting the drugs he would stop them. We accepted his plan not knowing what else to do.

The kidney transplant took as long as the liver transplant. When Dr. Goggins came out to discuss the surgery, he looked very tired. He had tried to place the kidney on her left side, but the artery he needed to use for the kidney could not be used. It had a blockage in it. So, he closed that side and opened her back up on the other side. He had not wanted to place the kidney beside the liver but felt he had no other choice. In addition, her abdominal muscles were very rigid from all the surgeries over the years; thus, he had to place a mesh inside her abdomen in order to close her up.

Even though the surgery had been one of the most difficult ones ever performed, he was pleased with how things had gone. The kidney had started working immediately. He stopped the dialysis that had been running continuously since the liver transplant. Typically, dialysis continues at least until the patient gets back to their room. Since the new kidney had been on a pump for three days while waiting, it usually took a while for it to be at full strength in the body. This kidney, however, was ready to start right up!

After Amy was taken back to her room in the Transplant ICU, she remained on a ventilator. The nurse said she would stay on it probably through the day and night. Amy, always full of the unexpected, was off it by evening.

Having her abdomen opened three times in as many days, Amy was in more pain than after the liver transplant. Over the following few days, her lab work showed the kidney to be working well.

By March 19, she had developed a urinary tract infection as well as thrush in her mouth which caused much mouth pain and kept her from eating. On Sunday, Michael and I went to church while Matt stayed with her. Just as church started, I received a text message from Matt telling me to call him right away. I got up from the service and left the sanctuary to call. The doctor said Amy was losing blood flow to her abdomen. He thought it was due to all the surgeries Amy had endured, both recently and in the past years. I was concerned it might mean the antirejection drugs were affecting the blood flow as it had done before in her feet and legs.

They would just watch it. It could turn around or might get worse. If it got worse, Amy might need skin grafts to her abdomen. I didn't know what would happen if the problem was related to the drugs. I let Michael know what was going on. When Pastor Mark called for people to come up for healing prayer, Michael went to the alter and got a prayer cloth for Amy.

After church, I went to the hospital. I wanted to see what Amy's abdomen looked like myself. Her skin was very red and had a large area that was turning purple. Matt said that area concerned the doctor the most. I gave Amy the prayer cloth asking her to tell the blood vessels to open and do their job.

The following day, Amy began to have difficulty swallowing. She had issues in the past requiring her esophagus to be stretched. I wondered if this was happening again. She also was constipated. Over the next few days, the problems kept getting worse.

On March 25th, an N/G tube was placed in Amy's nose and down into her stomach to keep it emptied as the doctors attempted to rectify the constipation problem. We also learned her creatinine had risen to 1.5 from 0.6. The doctors didn't know if this meant rejection, reoccurrence of oxalate damage to the kidney or what might be wrong. They decided to do a kidney biopsy. Dr. Goggins did not want to do a regular needle biopsy. He felt a need to open her up for the biopsy. Amy returned to surgery to be opened back up for the fourth time. With it being Friday, I figured we would have a long weekend waiting on the results.

When Amy had her first kidney transplant as a 15 month old, her creatinine had started rising within the first week of the transplant. The crystals had started destroying the kidney quickly. The fear this was repeating kept trying to enter my mine. I refused to accept it! I was determined to believe and have the faith that something else was going on, and the doctors could correct it. The doctors said her antirejection drug levels were high which might explain the elevated creatinine. I hoped it was that simple!

On Saturday, Amy's creatinine had come down to 1.3 which the unit doctor said was a good sign. The constipation was improving, so the doctor removed the N/G tube. Amy was so happy. She hated it! With it down, she couldn't concentrate on anything else. As the constipation was resolved, her swallowing improved. All day, we waited for the biopsy results but kept hearing they were not available.

On Sunday morning, Michael and I went to church. Our church family had been really good. They stood by Amy with support, prayers and faith that she would be healthy. We still didn't have any news to tell them about the biopsy results which everyone wanted to know. Once church started, Matt sent me a text message. The doctor had been in with the results, no rejection and no oxalate in the kidney! Her creatinine was down to 0.9. We along with our church family were elated.

During the time Amy was recovering from her transplant surgeries, Matt's grandmother passed away. He returned to Ohio for her funeral. We stayed in touch.

On Monday, Mar 28th, the doctors decided the dialysis port Amy had for the past two and a half years could be removed. The kidney was working well. Her creatinine was 0.7. For some reason, Amy was anxious about having it removed. Without it, she would have to be stuck every day for blood draws. She was in tears.

"Amy, you don't need it. Removing it is another step toward you being normal and healthy," I explained.

I reminded her that she had always been stuck for blood draws and had always handled it well. Finally, she calmed down and realized it would be nice to be free of the catheter in her chest.

The doctor explained exactly how he would remove it and reassured her there would not be any pain. He would make her aware of each step. The procedure itself took just a few minutes. Afterwards, Amy was glad it was out. Since she had lived and depended on that catheter for so long, she may have felt it was actually a part of her while not wanting to lose another piece of herself.

After the procedure, I took a picture of Amy with her gown pulled back so the area where the catheter had been was showing. I sent the picture to Matt to figure out what was missing. He immediately noticed the catheter was gone.

As Amy slept after the procedure, I had a chance to think about the previous two and a half weeks. I realized that not once did anyone seem concerned about the liver. There seemed to be a complete peace about the liver. Even I, who had not wanted Amy to have a liver transplant, felt so peaceful. I knew that God's hand was in it. I don't know why He didn't just perform a miraculous healing like we wanted, but this was His way. It would be okay!

Amy was discharged from the hospital on April 1st. She was happy to be back home but knew it would be at least another three months before she could return to Ohio with Matt and Joshua. Her abdomen was better. The blood flow was slowly returning. There were three new long suture lines and a smaller one from the biopsy surgery. She was sore and in a wheelchair but had confidence of being back on her feet soon.

She had to return to clinic at the hospital twice a week to see the doctors and have her blood drawn. On April 7th, an ultrasound was done on her left leg because it was extremely swollen and painful. A large blood clot was discovered. Amy was readmitted to the hospital for IV anticoagulant medications. She remained there for another five days until being discharged. We continued attending clinic twice a week.

By June, Amy was up walking with her prosthetics. Her liver and kidney were working perfectly. When she saw her transplant surgeon at the clinic one day, he stated that her labs could not be better, that when looking at them it appeared she had been born with that liver.

I don't know why Amy became so ill again and had to tolerate what she did. Life always seems to throw curves at us, and we find ourselves walking a different path than the previous one. One thing is for sure, we must keep our faith that God will deliver us from the evil attacking us. We don't know what the future holds, but we are expecting great things. We are who we are today because of Amy's journey. Watching our daughter suffer was hell on Earth. There were moments, our faith would waver, but those were the moments that drove us to our knees!

Concluding Remarks

As October 2016 comes to an end, I am sitting in my kitchen attempting to put words on paper. The air is cool and the leaves are starting to fall from the trees creating a colorful blanket across my back yard, something I was unable to appreciate the past three years.

Amy has returned to Ohio to live with Matt and Joshua. That is where she needs to be, with her husband and son. Three years was too long to wait, but we are grateful it wasn't longer.

Those three years were an extreme test of our faith. In the middle of the test, we wondered at times if we would ever see an end to it, the end we prayed for, Amy healthy and able to continue with her life. I wondered if I could remain strong enough to help Amy get there. God is good, and He brought us through attack after attack.

There is so much to be thankful for. My husband, Michael, stayed in this fight with us. Our marriage had been a struggle since Amy was born. Michael was always pushed aside as I used my energy for Amy, but he remained steadfast and helped Amy and Katie become wonderful God-focused young women. I know he will do the same for our younger daughters, Gabriella and Jaelynn. I love you.

Thank you, Matt, for being the husband you are to Amy. Some men would have turned tail and run from a wife as ill as Amy, but you stayed and supported her in so many ways.

Thank you Dr. Roese, Dr. Christy, Dr. Hladik and staff at the Columbus Regional Hospital and the Columbus Wound

Center, Indiana University Medical Center doctors and staff, Hope Volunteer Fire Department, Pastors Mark and Dona Owings, and Faith Victory Church members. There are so many people we are thankful for who have been there for us during this journey. It would be impossible to name them all!

Thank you David Webster. Without you, this book would not be a reality. You have worked so hard to see that all the i's were dotted and the t's were crossed. You are a blessing.

When we started this journey, it was to save Amy. Now that Amy is healthy again, I realized I needed saved too. Thank you, Amy, for leading me into a life of trust, forgiveness and faith.

Our entire family has realized we can trust in God. Even if things don't go the way we desire, God will be there and things will still be okay if we keep our faith.

Following is a word from Julie Bertarelli of The Oxalosis and Hyperoxaluria Foundation. Please take a moment to read what she has to say.

Today, there is a place to turn to for HOPE! The Oxalosis and Hyperoxaluria Foundation (OHF) was founded in 1989 thanks to the care, interest and actions of concerned parents and families, frustrated, confused and not sure where to turn after discovering that a loved one was diagnosed with a rare genetic disorder call Primary Hyperoxaluria (PH).

The families searched for hope, encouragement and information regarding PH. Together everyone pooled their time, talent and resources to find answers about this rare disease. They formalized a small group of families, physicians and researchers and eventually established the OHF. The OHF funded Mayo Clinic Hyperoxaluria Center which continues to be the leader in the world searching for a better treatment and cure for PH.

Please support our efforts in honor of Amy Lawson Steward to support this foundation so that one day no one will have to suffer the effects of this disease. To make a donation in honor of Amy, you may go to ohf. org for more information or mail to OHF, 201 East 19th Street, Suite 12E, New York, NY 10003.

Amy's Thanksgiving Plate

Throughout my life, I have referred to a plate that Amy Lawson made for our Thanksgiving bulletin board when she was in my fifth grade classroom in 1994. During that year, she had to fight for her life once again at Mayo Clinic in Minnesota. While reflecting about Amy's plate during her hospital stay, I was inspired to write a song. Another former student who was an excellent boxer, Corky Lonaker, gave me some reassuring words when talking to him about Amy. I consequently incorporated what he stated at the end of the song. Corky has certainly had his ups and downs since that day, in particular when losing his dad in a tragic accident in 2016. At the funeral home, we talked about his words in 1994. He assured me the fighter within would be a key in helping him through their family tragedy and in moving forward too. His dad would very much want it that way, someone who had helped him develop as a boxer.

David Webster

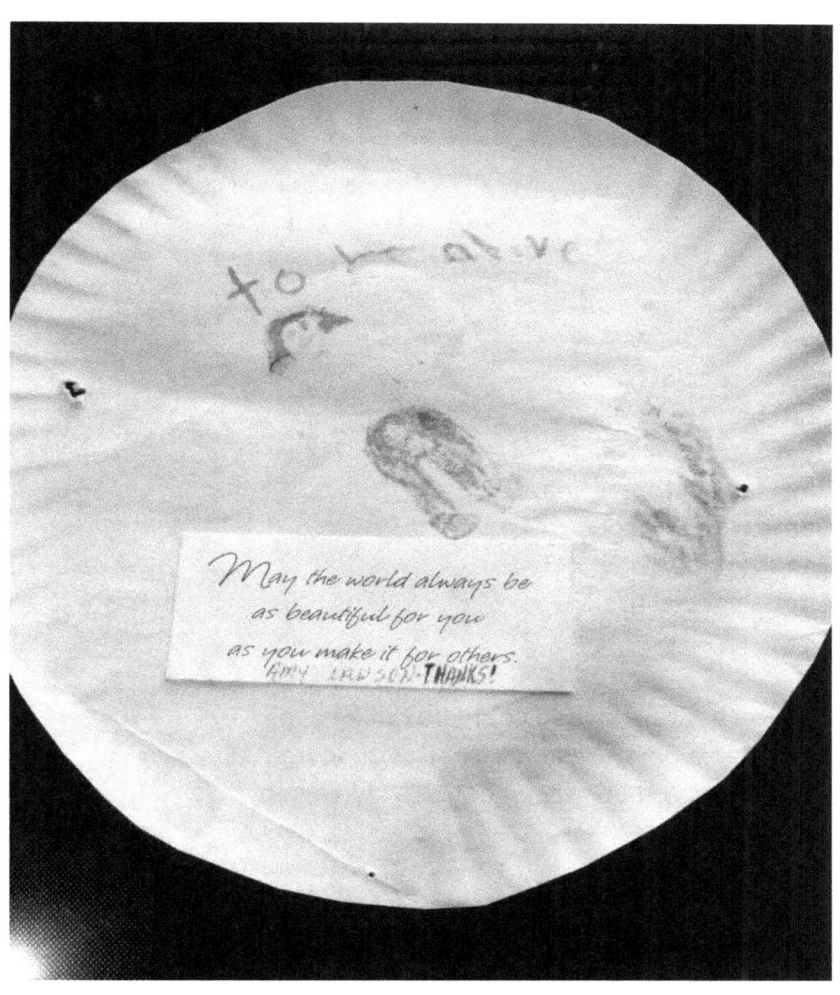

A Fighter Like You © 1994 by David Webster & Sally Webster

Walked into the classroom on the bulletin board
A Thanksgiving plate made by Amy
Thanking God for her life
Now I pray for you my friend

Chorus
God
Amy is special to us
Watch over her
Heal with your touch
Amy sees with her heart
Hears with her soul
Cannot depart
Amy is special to us

Kept on hearing kidney could be failing again
Years ago a parent gladly gave it with love
Sick and scared and flying her to Mayo again

Chorus

Met up with a boxer former student of mine
We started talking about you he said most of the time
A fighter like you will win again and again

Chorus

www.ingramcontent.com/pod-product-compliance
Lightning Source LLC
Chambersburg PA
CBHW062201280526
45788CB00001B/394